Nursing Care Planning Guides
Set 5

Margo Creighton Neal, RN, MN
VICE PRESIDENT, WILLIAMS & WILKINS

Patricia Feltz Cohen, RN, MA, EdM
CONSULTANT, HUNTINGTON BEACH, CA

Joan Reighley, RN, MN
PSYCHOTHERAPIST, PRIVATE PRACTICE, LOS ANGELES, CA
Certified, specialist; Division of Psychiatric and Mental Health Nursing,
American Nurses' Association

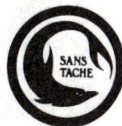

WILLIAMS & WILKINS
Baltimore • London • Los Angeles • Sydney

Contributors   Bettie Lilley Nosek, RN, BA
Ann Schofield, RN, MSN

Copyright © 1981—Margo Creighton Neal
Copyright © 1985- –Williams & Wilkins
428 East Preston Street, Baltimore, Maryland 21202 U.S.A.

Printed in the United States of America

Library of Congress Cataloging in Publication Data

Main entry under title:
Nursing care planning guides, set 5.

   1. Nursing—Handbooks, manuals, etc. 2. Nursing—Planning—Handbooks, manuals, etc. I. Neal, Margo Creighton, 1935–
II. Cohen, Patricia Feltz, 1932–   . III. Reighley, Joan, 1936–   . IV. Title.
RT51.N373   1981   610.73   81-16944
ISBN 0-683-09523-4

   86 87 88 89   10 9 8 7 6 5 4

Set No. 5
TABLE OF CONTENTS

INTRODUCTION

To use these Guides to greatest advantage, scan the Table of Contents and select the Guide that is related to a specific patient, for example, "The Patient with Addison's Disease." Note its separate components: long-term goal, general considerations, specific considerations, patient outcomes, nursing actions, discharge planning, and recommended references. Review other *Nursing Care Planning Guides* that have been recommended as relating to this content area: "Drugs: Corticosteroids" and "Teaching Patients: General Suggestions." If your patient has a behavior that requires nursing intervention, such as depression, review that guide also.

After this process, assess your patient in terms of the reviewed data, the presenting complaints, signs and symptoms, and behavior. Extrapolate from the Guides essential data that can help you with the next step in the nursing process—making the nursing diagnosis. The "Specific Considerations" section of the Guides contains general areas of nursing diagnosis, such as "Control of Symptoms" in "The Patient with Addison's Disease." To make the diagnosis, choose those specific symptoms/problems that are interfering with the patient's adjustment/recovery, such as weakness, fatigue; the latter become the nursing diagnosis. Next, specify expected outcomes for the nursing diagnosis, referring to those suggested in the Guide, using or changing them as appropriate. Expected outcomes, also known as goals or objectives, define *WHAT* you and the patient are trying to do about the nursing diagnosis (also known as the patient problem). Make as many nursing diagnoses, with corresponding outcomes, as necessary. If possible, set a long-term goal; sometimes this cannot be done until the results of diagnostic tests are in.

Next, prescribe nursing actions that will lead to the patient achieving the expected outcomes. Nursing actions define *HOW* you will achieve the outcomes. Refer to those suggested in the Guides and extrapolate accordingly; add additional ones based on your own nursing judgement. Set a timeframe for evaluating patient response to these interventions: is the patient moving toward the expected outcomes? If not, do you need to review the nursing actions? the outcomes? or is some other nursing diagnosis taking priority? If "yes" to any of these, then revise the plan as needed.

Consider discharge planning for your patient. What does your patient need to know on discharge? Incorporate this teaching into your nursing care plan.

Set 5 is cross-referenced to the four previously published sets of *Nursing Care Planning Guides.*

The Patient with Addison's Disease

Definition: Addison's Disease is primary adrenocortical insufficiency resulting in an inadequate supply of cortisol.

LONG TERM GOAL: The patient will reach and maintain the optimum level of performance possible, living within the limits of the disease and treatment regimen, preventing crisis medical emergencies; the patient will resume normal home, family, and community roles.

General Considerations:
- Thomas Addison first described this chronic, progressive disorder in 1855.
- **Incidence and occurrence:** approximately 4 per 100,000, all age groups, both sexes, but more common in women.
- **Causes:** idiopathic atrophy of adrenal cortex (likely caused by autoimmune diseases) comprises more than 70% of cases; other causes include tuberculous granuloma, necrosis, metastases, fungus infection.
- One patient in five may also be diabetic; other endocrine disorders may be associated with Addison's Disease as well as non-endocrine disorders of pernicious anemia and vitiligo (hypopigmented skin areas).
- **Signs and symptoms:** weakness, general malaise, fatiguability, anorexia, weight loss and other gastrointestinal disorders, hypotension, and hyperpigmentation. Diffuse tanning (especially of pressure points, skin folds, scars, etc.) occurs only in primary adrenal dysfunction because of excessive secretion of ACTH by the continuously-secreting pituitary gland trying to correct deficient levels of circulating cortisol. ACTH resembles the melanocyte-stimulating hormone. Parodoxically, idiopathic destruction of melanin-producing tissues can also cause patchy vitiligo.
- **Clinical findings** are related to the loss of sufficient adrenal cortex steroids. Cortisol deficiency leads to severe hypoglycemic reactions because of inability to maintain an adequate blood glucose level and because of the loss of the anti-insulin effect of cortisol. This produces fatigue and muscle aches due to lack of muscle and hepatic glycogen stores. A loss of mental acuity is also related. Insufficient cortisol leads to decreased secretion of gastrointestinal digestive enzymes causing a variety of GI disorders: nausea, vomiting, diarrhea, anorexia, abdominal cramps. Mineralocorticoid deficiency leads to potassium retention, hyperkalemia, and cardiac dysrhythmias as well as sodium wasting, hyponatremia, and depletion of extracellular fluid volume.
- In the presence of severe infection, injury, an operation, or other stressful event, exaggerated physical findings may lead to a physiological collapse known as **Addisonian Crisis**, a true medical emergency leading to shock and death if not promptly and correctly treated. Aggresive replacement of fluids, electrolytes, and exogenous glucocorticoids reverse dramatically this event.
- **Diagnosis** includes complete physical examination for additional underlying or associated diseases, laboratory procedures

involving baseline, plasma cortisol determinations, 24 hour urinary 17-hydroxycorticosteroids, quick or long method ACTH stimulation tests, and various arteriography studies.

— **Treatment and nursing responsibilities** involve control of symptoms with exogenous steroids replacement therapy, management of associated diseases, and a comprehensive patient education program.

Specific Considerations, Potential Patient Outcomes, and Nursing Actions:

1) Control of Symptoms

The patient's disease symptoms are reduced or controlled; the patient maintains nutrition and adequate weight; the patient is free of preventable complications;

— plan nursing care, tests, & teaching to allow for regular meals, rest periods & snack periods; know that pt. feels slightly stronger in AM, but will tire easily; give ample assistance & encouragement;

— determine which foods are best liked & tolerated; arrange for conducive environment for eating;

— know that pt. is unable to tolerate fasting due to hypoglycemia; to avoid a crisis, IV glucose & increased maintenance doses of steroids must be given prior to surgery or diagnostic procedures; explain reason to pt. & family;

— closely monitor daily I&O, weight; record vital signs Q4H, taking apical-radial pulse counts; institute cardiac monitoring for irregularities; be alert for postural hypotension; check BP before & after activity & position changes; explain to pt. need to change positions slowly & carefully;

— be alert for episodes of extreme weakness, abdominal pain, confusion, fever, or associated electrolyte imbalance signs; notify MD STAT as acute Addisonian Crisis may be impending; have IV cut-down supplies & 5% Dextrose in N/S ready for immediate administration; know that dexamethasone or hydrocortisone will probably also be ordered & have injectable form available;

— administer daily steroids as ordered, explaining this drug adminisration to pt. & family; teach pt. how to inject self IM for emergency needs; refer to NCPG #5:43, "Drugs: Corticosteroids" for side effects & nursing implications.

2) Psychosocial Adjustments

The patient demonstrates a productive, self-reliant adjustment to Addison's Disease and its management; the patient and family express feelings of acceptance, self-confidence, and alleviation of fear concerning lifelong condition:

— see NCPGs #1:44, "Suggestions for Interviewing," #1:49, "Teaching Patients: General Suggestions," & #5:30, "The Patient Adapting to Chronic Illness Role;"

— observe family relationships to estimate degree of support available to pt. after discharge; consider enlisting the aid of a friend PRN;

— explain to pt./family/significant other the nature of pt.'s condition & symptoms, the reason for lifelong steroid replacement therapy, & how to prevent an Addisonian Crisis; provide pt. with identification card & emergency medication kit with doctor's prescription;

— know, & explain to pt./family, that emotional upsets & tension increase need for steroids; attempt to determine & alleviate causes of stress & help pt. to cope more effectively with it; provide opportunities for pt./family to express feelings, concerns, frustrations & annoyances; refer to NCPG #5:49, "Stress Management," for additional information.

Discharge Planning and Teaching Objectives/Outcomes

1) (Patient/Family/Significant Other) Can explain own condition, symptoms, treatment, and prognosis.

1) Will keep a record of weight, drink plenty of fluids, and try to avoid occasions of undue physical exertion or emotional upset.

3) Can correctly demonstrate self IM injections and care of equipment without contamination.

4) Can tell the actions and side effects of steroids s/he is taking; has an adequate supply to take home and knows where and when to obtain refills. States s/he knows how to adjust drug dosage during times of physical or emotional stress.

5) Has a medical identification card, necklace, or bracelet and will wear at all times; will carry with self at all times an emergency drug kit (disposable syringes & needles, oral & injectable cortisol, doctor's letter of need & instructions for emergency use).

Recommended References

"Acute Adrenal Insufficiency," by Manuel Tzagournis. *Heart & Lung*, July-August 1978: 603-609.

"Adrenal Insufficiency," by Neil Schimke. *Critical Care Quarterly*, September 1980: 19-27.

"Drugs: Corticosteroids." *NCP Guide #5:43*, Nurseco, 1981.

"Dysfunction of the Adrenal Glands," by Sarah Sanford. *The Nursing Clinics of North America*, September 1980: 481-498.

"Interviewing: Suggestions for." *NCP Guide #1:44*, 2nd Ed., Nurseco, 1981.

"The Patient Adapting to Chronic Illness Role." *NCP Guide #5:30*, Nurseco, 1981.

"Stress Management." *NCP Guide #5:49*, Nurseco, 1981.

"Systems of Life No. 57 The Adrenal Glands — Disorders of Glucocorticoids," by Anne Roberts and Audrey Besterman. *Nursing Times*, September 20, 1979: 75-78.

"Teaching Patients: General Suggestions." *NCP Guide #1:49*, 2nd Ed., Nurseco, 1980.

"What's Wrong With Ellen?" by Catherine Garofano, *Nursing 80*, 1980: 98-99.

The Patient with Alzheimer's Disease

Definition: Alzheimer's Disease is a progressive deterioration in intellectual functioning due to cellular degeneration and formation of "senile plaques" in the cerebral cortex.

LONG TERM GOAL: The patient will be maintained for as long as possible in a state of bio/psycho/social integrity in a comfortable and protected environment; the family/significant other will receive information and emotional support.

General Considerations:

— Alzheimer's Disease is the major cause of severe organic brain dysfunction in older people and accounts for 50% of senile dementias; it is a strong factor in an additional 24%.

— **Prognosis** is poor with eventual breakdown of intellect and personality until the person is totally dependent on others; bowel and bladder control diminishes and the patient becomes like an infant. Death usually results from cardio-vascular, pulmonary, or renal complications.

— **Cause** is unknown. Theories include deficiency of acetylcholine leading to degeneration of presynaptic nerve terminals, formation of amyloid senile plaques by immunologic mechanism, slow-acting viruses, aluminum acting as a cytoxic factor, and genetic factors.

— **Onset** is insidious and may begin at any time from thirties to old age.

— **Symptoms** may include disturbed memory function, failure of perception, and decline in intellectual functioning. Patient seems unaware of any changes in mental functioning and cannot understand why others are concerned about them. Many elderly persons with Alzheimer's Disease become like good children and are amiable and cooperative. Twenty percent have paranoid reactions; as they begin to lose ability for insight and self-evaluation, they lose the ability to perceive self and others realistically. Suspicion, hostility, and hallucinations may occur.

— **Diagnosis** is usually made via mental status exam, symptoms, and history of onset of symptoms; EEG and laboratory tests may be done for borderline cases or to rule out other diagnosis.

— **Treatment** is symptomatic with no effect on the underlying disease. Faulty circulation through atherosclerotic blood vessels may also be present but is *not* the cause of cellular degeneration and formation of "senile" plaques. Therefore, no improvement is usually found with vasodilator or neurotransmitter drugs.

— **Nursing responsibilities** include recognition of symptoms of onset of Alzheimer's Disease, assessment and interventions to maintain bio/psycho/social integrity in a comfortable and protected environment, and offering information and emotional support to the family and significant other (SO).

Specific Considerations, Potential Patient Outcomes, and Nursing Actions:

1) Maintenance of Adequate Biophysical Status (Within Age and Disease Limitations)

The patient performs some activities of daily living (ADL) with minimal necessary assistance, maintains normal warm, moist skin and mucous membranes; has a minimum intake of 1500ml/day and an ouput of at least 900ml/day; attains and maintains desired weight; has at least one bowel movement every four days; attains and maintains ambulation with assistance as necessary; participates in exercise and rest periods daily; sleeps at least six hours nightly (preferably without sedation); has clear lungs and normal vital signs; is supervised for medication need and responses to medication and treatments:

— know that some pts. with Alzheimer's Disease also have nutritional deficiencies from poor intake or side effects from medications for other problems, i.e., high blood pressure, edema, heart disease; a well-balanced diet & vitamin supplements will avoid behaviors due to inadequate potassium, vitamin B_{12}, or folic acid;

— assess medications ordered for drugs known to lower serum folate levels such as barbiturates, phenytoin, primidone, phenylbutazone, nitrofurantoin, some analgesics, & possibly phenothiazines (Mellaril, Thorazine, Compazine, Phenergan); these drugs are contraindicated for persons with Alzheimer's Disease unless a folic acid supplement is taken; know that alcohol also lowers serum folate levels & should be used sparingly.

— for additional nursing actions, see NCP Guide #4:34, "The Aged Patient: Chronic Organic Brain Syndrome."

2) Maintenance of Adequate Psychosocial Status (Within Age and Disease Limitations)

The patient regains and maintains contact with reality; is oriented to time/place/person; appears minimally withdrawn and apathetic, interacting voluntarily with others and with environment in socially-appropriate ways; makes some decisions and choices related to own care and activities; reminisces to integrate life experiences; the family/SO receives emotional support and information about disease process and prognosis:

— assess family/SO for stage of loss; offer to spend private time with them for the purpose of ventilation of feelings & concerns;

— know that your presence is comforting as the family/SO goes through the process of grief & mourning for their previously normal, mentally-intact loved one who is now deteriorating mentally & must be cared for in special ways; accept their feelings in their time of actual loss, as the pt. is diagnosed & plans are made for long-term care, & as they anticipate the gradual deterioration in intellectual functioning & finally, death; see NCPGs #1:31, "Responses to Loss: The Grief & Mourning Process" & #5:30, "The Patient Adapting to Chronic Illness Role;"

— assess family/SO's knowledge of the disease process & prognosis; clarify information & health teach as needed; help them to understand & accept the pt.'s behavior;

— problem solve with them to discover ways in which they can visit & support pt. such as spending time reading to pt., bringing in photographs or family albums, & sharing appropriate hobbies or interests with pt.; see NCPG #5:47, "Problem Solving;"

— know that a stable environment with warm acceptance will help pt. achieve optimal functioning within the limitations of the disease process; interview family/SO to identify usual schedule, preferences, & adaptive coping mechanisms previously used by pt.; utilize these as much as possible in ADL; use environmental manipulation to assist pt. to cooperate with plan for ADL & activities, i.e., make dining room a warm & inviting place with plants, pets such as birds or fish, soft music, art objects, bulletin boards, round tables with opportunity for socialization & conversation during meals; let pt. use toilet articles brought from home, play soft music or relaxation tapes at rest or bedtime, put daily schedule & clock in each pt.'s room, giving positive reinforcement with praise, smiles, & rewarding experiences for cooperation in ADL & activities; see NCPGs #5:37, "Behavior Modification" & #5:32, "The Patient Experiencing A Threat to Self-Esteem;"

— for additional nursing actions, see NCPG #4:34, "The Aged Patient: Chronic Organic Brain Syndrome," nursing actions #2.

Discharge Planning and Teaching Objectives/Outcomes

1) (Patient/Family/Significant Other) Expresses understanding of disease process, prognosis, and the medical regimen prescribed; recognizes need for ongoing care in a comfortable and protected environment.

2) Has name and telephone number of attending physician, available community resource groups, social worker for financial and insurance help, and a mental health counselor for crisis and coping with chronic illness situation.

Recommended References

"The Aged Patient: Chronic Organic Brain Syndrome." *NCP Guide #4:34*, Nurseco, 1978.

"The Aged Patient: Common Behaviors." *NCP Guide #2:26*, 2nd Ed., Nurseco, 1980.

"The Aged Patient: Physiology of Aging." *NCP Guide #2:33*, 2nd Ed., Nurseco, 1980.

"The Aged Patient: Transition to Communal Living." *NCP Guide #2:2* 2nd Ed., Nurseco, 1980.

"Assessment of Mental Status." *NCP Guide #4:41*, Nurseco, 1978.

"Behavior Modification." *NCP Guide #5:37*, Nurseco, 1981.

"Coping with Impaired Brain Function," by Elaine Pasquali et al. *Mental Health Nursing.* St. Louis: C.V. Mosby Co., 1981:565-603.

Drugs and the Aged by William D. Poe & Donald A. Holloway. New York: McGraw-Hill Book Co., 1980: 70-86.

"The Patient Adapting to Chronic Illness Role." *NCP Guide #5:30*, Nurseco, 1981.

"The Patient Experiencing a Threat to Self-Esteem." *NCP Guide #5:32*, Nurseco, 1981.

"Problem Solving." *NCP Guide #5:47*, Nurseco, 1981.

"Responses to Loss: The Grief & Mourning Process." *NCP Guide #1:31*, 2nd Ed., Nurseco, 1980.

The Patient with Angina

Definition: Angina pectoris is a clinical syndrome of sudden, sharp pain or pressure in anterior chest produced by insufficient coronary blood flow and subsequent myocardial hypoxia.

LONG TERM GOAL: The patient will express adequate knowledge of the cause and precipitating factors of angina pectoris; the patient will demonstrate appropriate management of chemotherapy regimen and activities of daily living (ADL) to cope with stress.

General Considerations:

— **Cause:** usually atherosclerotic heart disease that obstructs the major coronary artery.

— **Precipitating factors** include intense emotions, exertion, exposure to cold, sudden tenseness, eating a large heavy meal, and life stresses.

— **Pain** may be mild or severe and last 1-10 minutes; pain radiates from sternum to left pectoral region, left shoulder, neck, and jaw, and may include inner aspect of left arm to hand. Patient may experience extreme anxiety, break out in a sweat, and have sensation of tightness, pressure, choking, heaviness in chest, and numbness or weakness of arms, hands, and wrists. *NURSING ALERT:* If pain last longer than 10 minutes or nitroglycerine does not relieve it, suspect impending myocardial infarction and notify physician immediately.

— **Treatment** includes chemotherapy (nitroglycerine (glycerine trinitrate) sublingual tablets, 0.15-0.60 mg) and patient education to avoid precipitating factors, to stop physical activity when pain occurs, to mangage nitroglycerine intake, and to change living habits and attitudes to manage stress. (Reconstructive coronary artery surgery to replace or bypass obstruction may be considered; see NCPGs #4:06 and 7, "The Patient Undergoing Cardiac Surgery.")

— **Nursing responsibilities** include assessment for symptoms and prompt treatment of angina pain, and patient education as oulined above.

Specific Considerations, Potential Patient Outcomes, and Nursing Actions:

1) Pain and Chemotherapy   The patient stops activity and takes nitroglycerine as directed, upon recognizing angina pain; the patient experiences prompt relief of pain and decrease in anxiety; the patient demonstrates management of chemotherapy regimen:

    — when pain occurs, advise pt. to stop activity, to rest, & to take nitroglycerine as ordered;

    — decrease pt.'s anxiety by speaking in calm, quiet voice, & carrying out tasks in unhurried way; ask pt. to describe pain & talk about fears & concerns;

    — decrease environmental stimuli such as noise & tiring or annoying visitors;

    — observe & chart location & duration of pain, the circumstances preceding the attack, vital signs, changes in color or sweating, & pt.'s response to medication;

    — teach & supervise pt./family/significant other (SO) administration, dosage, action of nitroglycerine & other medications pt. is taking; refer to NCPG #2:37, "Drugs: Cardiac."

2) Patient/
   Family
   Education

The patient/family states basic facts about angina, chemotherapy management, and avoidance of precipitating stressors; the patient assesses and revises as necessary diet, exercise, attitudes, and living habits in order to reduce cardiac workload and stressors:

    — assess learner level of knowledge & readiness to learn; correct misconceptions & provide new information PRN; establish trust & mutual respect by attentive listening, calling pt./family by name;

    — ask pt. to identify activities or emotions that precipitate angina pain; teach to avoid those known to precipitate pain such as sudden exertion, exposure to cold, walking against wind, heavy meals, intense excitement, life stresses;

    — teach immediate response to angina pain: stop activity, take nitroglycerine as directed, & expect prompt relief; advise pt/family/SO to contact Dr. immediately if pain persists 10 minutes after taking nitroglycerine;

    — assess need for weight reduction to reduce cardiac workload & health teach PRN; have dietitian work with pt. as needed;

    — advise & support non-smoking; inform pt. that smoking produces tachycardia & raises blood presure, thus increasing workload of heart;

    — assess pt.'s participation in regular exercise; explain that a regular, graded-exercise program helps to exercise below pain threshold & increase cardiac circulation; help pt. work a program into his regular schedule;

    — assess attitudes & living habits for effect on stress levels; help pt. to manage stress effectively; see NCPG #5:49, "Stress Management;"

    — refer to NCPG #1:49, "Teaching Patients: General Suggestions."

Discharge Planning and Teaching Objectives/Outcomes

1) (Patient/Family/Significant Other) Can describe in own words cause of angina and treatment plan to prevent and manage angina pain; can state immediate response to angina pain.

2) Knows to notify physician if pain persists 10 minutes after taking nitroglycerine.

3) Describes ADL and life-style changes that will decrease cardiac workload and effects of precipitating factors, and that will maintain stress at a manageable level.

4) Knows actions and side effects of all medications prescribed.

Recommended References

"Angina. Teaching Your Patient How to Prevent Recurrent Attacks," by Christine Walton and Betsy Hammond. *Nursing 78*, February 1978:32-38.

"Drugs: Cardiac." *NCP Guide #2:37*, 2nd Ed., Nurseco, 1980.

"Helping the Client with Unstable Angina," by S. Gronim. *The American Journal of Nursing*, October 1978:1677-1680.

"Stress Management." *NCP Guide #5:49*, Nurseco, 1981.

"The Effect of Antianginal Drugs on Myocardial O_2 Consumption," by Ellen Fuller. *The American Journal of Nursing*, February 1980:250-254.

"The Patient Undergoing Cardiac Surgery." *NCP Guides #4:06, 07*, Nurseco, 1978.

"Variant Angina — a Nursing Approach," by R. Cain et al. *Heart and Lung*, November-December 1979:1122-1126.

"When Your Patient Has Chest Pain," by M. Rodman. *RN*, December 1980:43

The Patient Needing Angiography

Definition: Angiography is the roentgenographic visualization of blood vessel networks through intravenous or arterial injection of a radiopaque dye.

LONG TERM GOAL: The patient will derive full therapeutic benefit from diagnostic angiography and will accept and understand the course of action indicated by the procedure's results.

General Considerations:
— **Indications:** diagnostic verification of the diseases associated with the heart or cardiovascular system, kidneys and renal system, brain or ventricular system, and portal-caval or associated intra-abdominal vessel networks.
— Angiography procedures are usually performed in x-ray department by radiologist and technician. Percutaneous or cut-down approach for dye (contrast material) injection is often done.
— **Potential complications** associated with angiography include drug reactions to the dye such as dyspnea, nausea, vomiting, numbness of extremities, diaphoresis, tachycardia, and cardiac dysrhythmias.
— **Nursing responsibilities** include: (1) patient teaching/family counseling regarding procedural steps and likely outcomes; (2) obtaining an informed, signed, and witnessed consent record; and (3) close monitoring of patient for early or delayed onset of drug reaction and for injection site complications of bleeding or hematoma formation.

Specific Considerations, Potential Patient Outcomes, and Nursing Actions:

1) Pre-angiography Preparation of Patient

The patient's anxiety state is minimized; the patient understands the procedure, technique, equipment, potential risks, and expected side effects of the dye and drugs associated with angiography:
— assess pt.'s knowledge or misconceptions about the procedure; encourage free flow of questions/ answers until procedure is properly understood;
— orient pt. to angiography environment, equipment, & physical expectations during procedure; explain to pt./family/visitors that procedure may take 30' to 2 hrs.;
— inform pt. that the examination table may be tilted during the procedure to facilitate better exposure, that ECG leads may be attached to monitor cardiac response, & that s/he may be requested to cough, deep breathe or hold breath at intervals during procedure, but otherwise, to lie quietly;
— prepare pt. for various possible sensations normally experienced during dye injection, such as hot, flushing

effect with burning sensation along course of injected vessel, accompanied by slight discomfort at injection site or nausea or palpitations;
- obtained signed & witnessed written consent form;
- record complete, accurate vital signs, including peripheral pulses, to be used as a baseline for comparison with post-angiography vital signs;
- shave & cleanse proposed injection site; locate & mark on skin the peripheral pulse sites to facilitate nursing evaluation after procedure;
- ensure NPO status for 6-8 hrs. prior to procedure; give enema, if prescribed, to promote unobstructed radiographs;
- have pt. empty bladder just before giving prescribed sedation; record pt.'s reaction & condition just prior to leaving unit for x-ray.

2) Post-angiography Assessment and Care

The patient recovers from the angiography procedure free of preventable complications:
- instruct pt. that a period of restricted activity (bed rest, no BRP) must be observed following procedure; time may vary according to site of injection & pt.'s recovery response;
- encourage extension of extremity injection site to avoid increased pressure & potential hemorrhage; avoid elevation of legs, if pt. has a possible diagnosis of aortic aneurysm;
- observe for signs of numbness, pain, or bleeding in involved extremity & report accordingly; note skin color & temperature — compare with uninvolved extremity & record observation;
- monitor vital signs, record data, & report abnormalities; record I&O for 24 hrs.;
- inspect pressure dressing on insertion site for bleeding Q15min. until potential for hemorrhage is alleviated; use sandbags for extra pressure when indicated; observe also for hematoma formation at injection site; apply ice bags to reduce edema & discomfort;
- check pulses in the extremity distal to arterial insertion site Q15min. for 4 hrs. & note/report diminishing pulses;
- observe signs of drug reactions; be familiar & prepared for responsibilities related to treatment of acute drug reactions & anaphylactic shock;
- maintain an environment conducive to rest, following a naturally-fatiguing, anxiety-producing procedure.

Discharge Planning and Teaching Objectives/Outcomes
1) (Patient/Family/Significant Other) Demonstrates proper technique for care of injection site.

2) Understands and accepts outcome of diagnostic angiography and states s/he knows recommended course of action.
3) States s/he will observe and report potential complications of phlebitis such as painful redness or localized swelling at catheter/intravenous site.
4) Has confirmed physician appointment.

Recommended References

"Angiography in a Hurry." by A.J. Gerlock. Jr. *Emergency Medicine*. January 1979:243-244.
"How to See Your Patient Through an Angiogram." by Nancy Long. *RN*, October 1978:60-63.

The Patient with an Aortic Aneurysm

Definition: A localized, dilated area (*saccular,* not affecting entire circumference of vessel, or *fusiform,* involving entire circumference) of the thoracic or abdominal aorta. A dissecting type refers to one in which the vessel wall separates and blood is forced between layers: Type A involves the ascending aorta and Type B identifies those in the descending aorta.

LONG TERM GOAL: The patient will have condition stabilized in preparation for surgical intervention to repair aneurysm; the patient will recover from safe, successful resection of the aneurysm and return to usual roles in home, family, and community after a moderate convalescence; if inoperable due to critical condition, the patient will be sustained for as long as possible and the patient and family will be helped to cope with the crisis of loss.

General Considerations:

— **Signs and symptoms** vary according to patient and severity of aneurysm; patient may feel fit and without pain or may feel pain in upper abdomen or lumbar region; signs of hypertension present; hematemesis, bloody stools and/or N/V may be present if aneurysm is dissecting.

— **Etiology:** common among middle-aged males, contributing factors include: arteriosclerosis, trauma, congential vascular disease, or infection with necrosis of media vessel layer.

— **Diagnosis** is made by thorough physical examination and history; chest x-ray and follow-up angiography; vessels and aneurysm may also be visualized with ultrasound and/or computer tomography

— **Treatment:** prompt surgical resection with replacement of affected section by a Dacron or Teflon graft; surgery may be postponed depending on site (descending aorta) of aneurysm or patient condition (over 80, concomitant unrelated terminal illness or documented renal failure); medical management is similar to post-op management: aim to control blood pressure and to maintain respiratory, cardiovascular, renal, and neurological functions.

— **Nursing responsibilities:**

1) After consultation with attending physician, share with the patient/family/significant other the possibility of death; encourage them to express their feelings; provide crisis intervention; refer to NCPG #2:31, "The Patient Needing Crisis Intervention."

2) Provide system maintenance to meet treatment goals; intensive primary nursing care is usually needed. If aneurysm is dissecting type, admission may be to an ICU to stabilize patient's vital signs, monitor cardiac and renal output, and to control pain.

Specific Considerations, Potential Patient Outcomes, and Nursing Actions:

1) Preoperative Measures

The patient will have a determination of baseline values for post-op evaluation of circulatory status; the patient's aneurysm will be examined for location, size, and type; the patient will be prepared for successful surgery and will demonstrate post-op coughing and exercise routines:

— refer to NCPG #5:02, "The Patient With Angiography;" reinforce what pt. has been told about procedure; provide explanation PRN;

— monitor & record vital signs; check for bruits in femoral arteries; record peripheral pulse readings (dorsalis pedis) both legs;

— query for amt. of cigarette smoking, allergies, other illness, & medications; record results of physical exam, including palpation of abdomen, evidence of impaired circulation of extremities; NOTE: avoid elevating legs because pressure on aneurysm increases risk of rupture;

— have pt. indicate understanding of post-op routine, importance of coughing, ability to perform plantar flexion leg exercises; assure pt. that adequate pain med. will be given; provide time to answer pt./family questions & assuage fears;

— refer to NCPG #2:44, "General Preoperative Care;" care is similar to those having general abdominal surgery: an NG tube is placed, standard skin prep is done; continuous IV fluids are given & a CVP line is placed; refer to NCPGs #2:46, "Intravenous Therapy," #2:40, "Central Venous Pressure Line," & #5:46, "Nasogastric Intubation."

2) Post-operative Measures

The patient maintains adequate cardiopulmonary, elimination, musculoskeletal and other normal body functions; the patient maintains adequate fluid and electrolyte balance, normal gastrointestinal function is restored and the patient tolerates and progresses to a normal diet; the patient is free of preventable complications of hemorrhage, renal failure, pneumonia, and thrombophlebitis:

— refer to NCPGs #2:41, 42, 43, "General Postoperative Nursing Care, Part A, Part B, Part C;"

— maintain relatively flat position for about a week, avoiding extreme flexion which would increase abdominal pressure & impair leg circulation;

— check dressings for excess blood or drainage; use abdominal binder to provide support & comfort for moving or coughing;

— record vital signs as frequently as ordered, reporting changes; monitor & record dorsalis pedis pulses at same times;

— record I&O carefully & accurately; report dropping output of 30 ml. or less;

— give ice chips while NPO; after bowel sounds return & pt. is allowed oral fluids, note amt. & tolerance; progress to regular diet as ordered & tolerated;
— note & report post-op back pain as it may be a sign of retroperitoneal hemorrhage or a thrombus developing at graft site;
— note & report leg numbness or inability to move: it may be a sign of transient local edema exerting pressure on femoral nerve OR a developing arterial thrombus;
— encourage & monitor leg exercises at least Q2-3H; remove & re-apply elastic stockings at least Q8H;
— give analgesics, sedatives, antibiotics, & other medications as ordered; observe for untoward reactions;

Discharge Planning and Teaching Objectives/Outcomes

1) (Patient/Family/Significant Other) Has written appointment, date and time for follow-up visit to surgeon.
2) States s/he knows what to expect re: length of convalescence (approximately 4-6 weeks), diet (to control hypertension), and care of operative site (soap and water cleansing; dry, sterile dressing). If taking medications home, knows what they are, indications, expected effects, dosage, and administration.
3) Knows not to sit for long periods (over 45 min.) without occasional light exercise (walking or leg exercises).
4) Knows to call doctor for signs of illness, abdominal distention or pain, fever, or breaking away of incision.

Recommended References

"Acute Aortic Dissection," by Ellen Bramoweth. *The American Journal of Nursing,* November 1980:2010-2012.
"Central Venous Pressure Line." *NCP Guide #2:40,* 2nd Ed., Nurseco. 1980.
"General Preoperative Nursing Care." *NCP Guide #2:44,* 2nd Ed., Nurseco. 1980.
"General Postoperative Nursing Care, Parts A, B, and C."*NCP Guides #2:41, 42, 43,* 2nd Ed., Nurseco. 1980.
"Intravenous Therapy." *NCP Guide #2:46,* 2nd Ed., Nurseco. 1980.
"Nasogastric Intubation: General Principles." *NCP Guide #5:46,* Nurseco, 1981.
"Patrick H.: A Patient With An Abdominal Aortic Aneurysm," by Sarah Cook. *RN,* March 1978:71-76.
"The Patient Needing Crisis Intervention." *NCP Guide #2:30,* 2nd Ed., Nurseco. 1980.
"The Patient With Angiography." *NCP Guide #5:02,* Nurseco. 1981.

The Patient with Colporrhaphy/Colpoplasty or A&P Repair

Definition: Colporrhaphy is suture repair of vagina; colpoplasty is a plastic operation upon vagina. Terms are used interchangeably, with the latter becoming popular in some places. More common is term A&P Repair which is anterior and posterior colporrhaphy done at same time.

LONG TERM GOAL: The patient will derive full benefit from successful colporrhaphy and will return to usual roles in home, job, community after a normal, short, uneventful convalescence.

General Considerations:
- **Types** of colporrhaphy include: *anterior*-surgical repair of a cystocele (a herniation or protrusion of the bladder into the vaginal wall): *posterior*-surgical repair of rectocele (a herniation or protrusion of the rectum into the vagina): and perineorrhaphy (surgical repair of pelvic floor).
- **Indications** for anterior colporrhaphy include signs of urinary stress incontinence associated with increased abdominal pressure caused by activities such as coughing, laughing, walking, or lifting. Others are repeated urinary infections, residual urine, pelvic pressure, and interference with sexual intercourse. Indications for posterior colporrhaphy include: rectal irritation, constipation, incontinence, and hemorrhoids that resist medical treatment. Indications for perineorrhaphy are a relaxation of pelvic musculature that results in colpocele (a fold of vaginal mucosa protruding outside the vaginal orifice). Pelvic or low back pain and discomfort associated with sexual intercourse are other reasons for surgical repair.
- **Treatment** may be limited to simple anterior colporrhapy, but often includes a combined A&P Repair along with a vaginal hysterectomy, if otherwise also indicated.
- **Nursing responsibilities** are similar to those of caring for a patient with a vaginal hysterectomy (see NCPG #1:12): provide the patient with the information and reassurance she wants or needs re: hospitalization, the surgery, the expected postoperative course, and convalescence.

Specific Considerations, Potential Patient Outcomes, and Nursing Actions:

1) Preoperative Measures   The patient describes the objectives and expected outcomes of her surgery; the patient assists with and receives appropriate preoperative care:
   - provide cleansing *douches* for anterior colporrhaphy & cleansing *enemas* for posterior colporrhaphy, as ordered;
   - provide skin prep & low-residue diet (to reduce perineal straining postoperatively) as ordered;

— suggest positions that will relieve tension on suture line postoperatively;

— explain post-op catheter care & other necessary routines (coughing, deep breathing);

— see NCPG #2:44, "General Preoperative Nursing Care," for additional considerations.

2) Post-operative Measures and Prevention of Complications

The patient maintains adequate cardiopulmonary, elimination, musculoskeletal and other normal body functions; the patient maintains adequate fluid and electrolyte balance, normal gastrointestinal function is restored, and the patient tolerates and progresses from a clear liquid to a normal diet; the patient is free of preventable complications of hemorrhage, infection, and venous thrombosis:

— provide perineal care to prevent wound infection using sterile equipment, solutions, & technique;

— position pt. in low Fowler's to prevent tension on taut suture lines & to reduce pelvic pressure, thus promoting pt. comfort;

— promote increased intake of fluids & monitor I&O; observe carefully because of urethral edema & nearby sutures; refer to NCPG #2:39, "Catheters: Indwelling, Urethral;" after catheter removal, check voiding Q4H; measure amts. voided; notify doctor if pt. voiding frequent, small amts. or if unable to void in 6 hrs. when intake has been adequate; observe for signs of bladder infection;

— turn, cough, & deep breathe pt. Q2H;

— remove & replace anti-embolic stockings or elastic bandages Q8H; provide passive (later, active) leg exercises for pt.;

— provide adequate pain relief PRN to promote pt. comfort;

— check vital signs according to standard post-op procedure; observe & record for signs of hemorrhage, infection, thrombosis or embolus;

— progress pt. on schedule according to orders & tolerance, from clear liquids to low residue diet (needed to prevent abdominal cramping, straining at stool, and intra-abdominal pressure on healing suture lines);

— discourage activities that reduce leg circulation, such as pillows under knees or elevated bed gatch, crossed legs, etc.; promote early ambulation to counteract venous stasis caused by lithotomy position in surgery;

— see NCPGs #2:41, 42, 43, "General Postoperative Nursing Care," for additional appropriate nursing measures.

Discharge Planning and Teaching Objectives/Outcomes

1) (Patient/Family/Significant Other) Demonstrates positive adaptation to self-care activities (self-confidence and demonstrated

knowledge and skills).

2) Knows to observe and report promptly potential complications encountered with suture breakdown and absorption (hemorrhage, sharp pain in area, foul-smelling discharge).

3) Knows to observe and report promptly potential complications associated with embolus or phlebitis (sudden chest pain, difficulty breathing, reddened & swollen areas in lower extremities or at IV sites.

4) Has written appointment for surgical follow-up visit; knows what to do re: diet, activity, and medications (time, dosage, side effects).

Recommended References

"Catheters: Indwelling. Utheral." *NCP Guide #2:39*. 2nd Ed.. Nurseco. 1980.
"General Postoperative Nursing Care, Part A, Part C." *NCP Guides #2:41, 42, 43*. 2nd Ed.. Nurseco. 1980
"General Preoperative Nursing Care." *NCP Guide #2:44*. 2nd Ed.. Nurseco. 1980.
"The Patient with a Hysterectomy." *NCP Guide #1:12*. 2nd Ed.. Nurseco. 1980.

The Patient with Cushing's Syndrome

Definition: Primary or adrenal Cushing's Syndrome is a disorder of adrenal cortex hypersecretion of cortisol. When adrenal hypersecretion is secondary to excessive pituitary secretion of ACTH, the condition is known as "pituitary Cushing's Disease."

LONG TERM GOAL: The patient will reach and maintain optimum level of performance possible, living within the limits of the disease and treatment regimen, preventing complications when possible; the patient will resume normal home, family, community roles.

General Considerations:

— **Occurs:** in both children and adults, ten times more common in females.
— **Causes:** tumor or hyperplasia of adrenal gland (more common in children) tumor of pituitary gland or tumors outside pituitary secreting ACTH (more common in adults); overadministration of exogenous glucocorticoids.
— **Signs and symptoms:** abnormal fat distribution (characterized by round, moon-face, "buffalo hump" fat pad on back of neck and between shoulder blades, abdominal and waist fat), centripetal hypertension, hyperglycemia, facial plethora (redness), hirsutism (abnormal facial and body hair), muscular weakness, menstrual irregularities, osteoporosis, glycosuria, bruises and purple striae, susceptibility to infection, cessation of linear growth in children and mood swings into nervous depression.
— **Diagnosis:** laboratory tests including serum electrolytes, glucose tolerance, blood ACTH levels, dexamethasone suppression test and urinary free cortisol levels; a plasma cortisol concentration determination at three different times in a 24-hour period (AM, PM and the third on the following morning after a midnight test dose of dexamethasone). For differentiating *adrenal* Cushing's Syndrome from *pituitary* Cushing's Disease and for determining exact location of lesion, a battery of x-rays are performed, including at least: computerized tomography, ultrasonography, IV renal pyelography, arteriography and venography, pneumoencephalography and skull x-rays.
— **Treatment:** For *adrenal* Cushing's Syndrome, an adrenalectomy (unilateral or bilateral) with temporary or permanent cortisol replacement therapy. For *pituitary* Cushing's Disease, a hypophysectomy or transphenoidal microresection of neoplasm with steroid replacement therapy; other options include cobalt irradiation for patients under twenty or chemotherapy for metastatic tumors or for those for whom an operation is not feasible. In these latter cases, there is some success reported for drugs cyproheptadine or aminoglutethimide. Management of associated diseases (one in four also have diabetes) and a comprehensive patient education program complete the treatment plan.

— **Nursing responsibilities** are those of assessment, planning, intervention, and evaluation in the assistance of the patient and family to accept, adapt and cope effectively with the symptoms, diagnostic tests, treatment program, and life-long steroid replacement regimen.

Specific Considerations, Potential Patient Outcomes, and Nursing Actions:

1) Control of Symptoms

The patient's disease symptoms are reduced or controlled; the patient maintains adequate nutrition and weight control; the patient is free of preventable complications:

— record weight daily; measure I&O accurately: monitor vital signs Q4H; record & report all changes;
— check urine at least BID for sugar & acetone; observe & report signs of hyperglycemia (flushed, dry skin, drowsiness, headache, fatigue, rapid pulse);
— observe & report signs of hypokalemia (general malaise, apathy, muscle cramps, mental confusion, dizziness on arising);
— give antacids with between meal medications; observe for hematemesis, melena;
— provide diet as prescribed, probably hi-pro, mod-CHO, lo-fat, lo-Na and high in Potassium; help pt. & family to learn about & accept dietary restrictions;
— maintain a protective, safety-conscious environment to prevent bruises, infections & pathological fractures; keep bed low with bed rails up; help pt. when getting up from bed or chair (be alert for signs of postural hypotension: dizziness);
— teach & maintain habits of good hygiene, skin care, & foot care;
— keep pt. mobile & active, providing a balance between rest & exercise;
— know that after surgical removal of disease cause, steroid replacement therapy will be prescribed; explain side effects & recommendded precautions to pt. & family; refer to NCPG #5:43, "Drugs: Corticosteroids" for additional information.

2) Psycho-social Adjustment

The patient demonstrates a productive, self-reliant adjustment to Cushing's Syndrome and its management; the patient and family express feelings of acceptance, self-confidence, and alleviation of fear concerning a life-long condition:

— explain need for many & varied diagnostic tests; explain procedure as well as purpose;

— know that significant alteration in body image creates numerous physical & mental health problems for pt.; establish empathic rapport with pt. & family; facilitate coping by encouraging a verbalization of feelings; offer explanations of physiological basis for these changes; refer to NCPG #2:29, "The Patient Experiencing a Body Image Disturbance" for additional suggestions;

— know that emotional disruptions ranging from suicidal depression to euphoria are common; help staff accept pt. & behavior/mood changes; help pt. & family cope with these changes by explanations, calm acceptance, compassionate concern; refer to NCPG #1:26 "The Patient Experiencing Depression" for additional suggestions;

— know that insomnia enhances mood intensities; promote calm, relaxing rest periods during day for pt. & help ensure night sleep with medications PRN as ordered;

— exhibit patience, understanding, & a desire to listen when pt. demonstrates euphoric & talkative behavior;

— observe & carefully record all pt. behavior responses.

Discharge Planning and Teaching Objectives/Outcomes

1) (Patient/Family/Significant Other) Can explain own condition, symptoms, treatment, and prognosis.
2) Will keep a record of weight, blood pressure, temperature, urine sugars, and a diary of responses to medication.
3) Can tell the actions and side effects of all medications s/he is taking; knows when, why, and how they are to be taken; has an adequate supply to take home.
4) Has a medical identification card, necklace, or bracelet and will wear at all times.
5) Recognizes importance of regular medical follow-up visits and has a plan for keeping all appointments.

Recommended References

"Cushing's Syndrome: A Tripartite Entity," by Ernest Gold. *Hospital Practice*, June 1979:67-75.

"Diet: Low Sodium." *NCP Guide #3:44*, Nurseco, 1977.

"Drugs: Corticosteroids." *NCP Guide #5:43*, Nurseco, 1981.

"Dysfunction of the Adrenal Glands." by Sarah Sanford. *The Nursing Clinics of North America*, September 1980:486-487.

"Frank's Condition — Is It Serious?" by Catherine Garofano. *Nursing 80*, April 1980:30-31.

"The Nature of the Endocrine System Part 4: The Adrenal Glands," by Kenneth Shaw. *Nursing Mirror*, June 9, 1977:32-35.

"The Patient Experiencing a Body Image Disturbance." *NCP Guide #2:29*, 2nd Ed., Nurseco, 1980.

"The Patient Experiencing Depression." *NCP #1:26*, 2nd Ed., Nurseco, 1980.

"The Patient with Osteoporosis." *NCP Guide #3:12*, Nurseco, 1977.

The Patient with a Gastrostomy

Definition: A gastrostomy is a temporary or permanent opening into the stomach in order to feed a patient and maintain adequate nutrition.

LONG TERM GOAL: The patient will recover from a safe, successful gastrostomy free of preventable complications; the patient will maintain adequate nutrition via a gastrostomy feeding tube; the patient will cope adaptively with body-image change and will assume responsibility for own enteral therapy, when able.

General Considerations:

— **Indications:** obstruction of esophagus or oral structures by benign or malignant lesions, trauma or scar tissue; defects in swallowing due to CVA, degenerative neuromuscular disease or severe organic brain syndrome; systemic disease causing profound anorexia and malnutrition. Gastrostomy avoids many of the problems associated with parenteral nutrition or complications of nasogastric tube.

— **Techniques** vary: under local anesthesia (usually), through an upper midline abdominal incision, a stomach mucosa "tube" is fashioned and sutured to abdominal wall; a stoma is created with cautery and through this artificial "fistula" a gastric catheter or feeding tube is inserted and secured. Tube feedings are begun two to three days after the surgery. Gastrostomy has been done for more than 130 years.

— **Complications** include: cardiac dysrhythmias, pulmonary embolus, aspiration pneumonia, gastric secretion leakage from stoma wound infection, peritonitis. Complications are more common in those aged patients who are debilitated or in an advanced stage of disease. Surgical and medical advances have made this operation safer and more satisfactory for patients.

— **Nursing responsibilities** include pre-op teaching specific to gastrostomy and body-image change, establishment of fluid and electrolyte balance and stable vital signs, a standard abdominal skin prep, cleansing enema, intestinal antibiotics and pre-op sedation, placement of a CVP line, continuous intravenous fluids and, if condition permits, passage of a nasogastric tube. Refer to NCPGs #2:44, "General Preoperative Nursing Care," #2:46, "Intravenous Therapy," #2:40, "Central Venous Pressure Line," #2:29, "The Patient Experiencing a Body Image Disturbance," and #5:46, "Nasogastric Intubation: General Principles."

Specific Considerations, Potential Patient Outcomes, and Nursing Actions:

1) Cardiopul-
   monary
   Function

The patient maintains adequate ventilation; the patient coughs up bronchial secretions; the patient has clear lungs and is free of atelectasis and pneumonia; the patient has efficient circulating blood volume and complications of hemorrhage and shock are prevented/controlled:
- refer to NCPG #2:41, Part A: "Support of Pulmonary Functions," & NCPG #2:42, Part B: "Support of Cardiovascular/Renal Functions;"
- turn, cough & deep breathe pt. Q2H; IPPB treatments may be given to stimulate deep breathing & mucus removal;
- check CVP line & record reading @ least hourly; monitor & record TRP & BP as ordered, noting quality & changes;
- check dressings for bleeding or gastric leakage; reinforce or replace sterile dressing as necessary; keep MD informed.

2) Fluids and
   Electrolyes

The patient maintains an optimum fluid and electrolyte balance; the patient has a satisfactory intake and output; the patient is free of preventable complications and imbalances:
- accurately monitor & record all fluid intake & output, carefully measuring solution used to irrigate NG or gastrostomy tube; estimate diaphoresis & wound drainage; measure urine & check for sugar & specific gravity;
- observe for fluid & electrolyte imbalance; refer to NCPGs #3:48 & 3:49, "Fluids & Electrolytes, Part A: Fluids, Part B: Electrolytes;"
- keep nasogastric tube patent, functioning & securely connected to low, intermittent suction; don't try to push, pull or reposition tube (in order to avoid injury to gastric suture line); irrigate tube with prescribed amt. of NS as ordered & needed, recording amt. used & returned on I&O record; note color & amt. of drainage (should be bright red turning to dark red after first 12- 24 hrs. post- op); report excessive bleeding & vomiting immediately;
- when ordered, irrigate gastrostomy tube gently with room temperature NS 20-50 ml. to assure patency, to remove clots, to detect fresh bleeding; gastrostomy feedings will usually be started when bowel function returns (note this) & suture line has healed sufficiently; see NCPG #5:50, "Tube Feedings: General Principles;"
- administer parenteral fluids, observing administration site for redness, infiltration, leakage;
- check bowel elimination; report diarrhea or constipation; take corrective measures.

3)	Infection Control	The patient is free of infections:

3) Infection Control

The patient is free of infections:
- note & report temperature elevations of two or more degrees 3rd PO day;
- administer antibiotics ordered with appropriate methods for effectiveness, checking literature & with pharmacist;
- use strict aseptic technique when handling dressings, drainage tubes & collection devices; apply antibiotic ointment & skin protective cream around stoma; keep sterile dressings dry; use abdominal binder for support, even when pt. is in bed.

4) Psychosocial Adjustment

The patient/family/significant other, (SO) adapts effectively to the trauma of surgery, the stress of hospitalization, the seriousness of disease condition; the patient/family/SO accepts a body image change of gastrostomy and the altered eating pattern necessitated; the patient/family/SO experiences relief of fears from lack of information and expresses growing ability to cope with patient's care upon discharge;
- administer analgesics liberally PRN, remembering individual needs & pain thresholds;
- assess psychological status of pt. & refer to appropriate nursing guides on behaviors observed; see NCPG #2:29, "The Patient Experiencing a Body Image Disturbance;"
- assess what pt./family/SO knows about pt.'s condition & health teach PRN; know that having information can counteract fear & anxiety;
- as recovery progresses & plans are made for discharge to home care or convalescent hospital, involve the pt., family, & friends; teach necessary information about administering medications, nutrition via gastrostomy tube; make apporpriate referrals for assistance PRN.

Discharge Planning and Teaching Objectives/Outcomes
1) (Patient/Family/Significant Other) Has written appointment date and time for follow-up visit with doctor; knows to report promptly any signs of infection, nausea, vomiting, diarrhea, abdominal cramping or distention, polyuria or excessive thirst.
2) Knows how to test urine for sugar and to report findings of glucosuria promptly to doctor.
3) Knows how to administer own tube feedings, medications, and other care using suitable precautions; has demonstrated competency in this procedure and expresses confidence in ability.
4) Has received appropriate community health and welfare assistance referrals.

Recommended References

"Central Venous Pressure Line." *NCP Guide #2:40,* 2nd Ed., Nurseco, 1980.

"Fluids & Electrolytes. Part A: Fluids, Part B: Electrolytes." *NCP Guides #3:48, 49,* Nurseco, 1977.

"General Postoperative Nursing Care, Part A: Support of Pulmonary Function, Part B: Support of Cardiovascular/Renal Functions & Part C: Support of Auxillary Functions." *NCP Guides #2:41, 42, 43,* 2nd Ed., Nurseco, 1980.

"General Postoperative Nursing Care." *NCP Guide #2:44,* 2nd Ed., Nurseco, 1980.

"Intravenous Therapy: General Principles." *NCP Guide #2:46,* 2nd Ed., Nurseco, 1980.

"Nasogastric Intubation: General Principles." *NCP Guide #5:46,* Nurseco, 1981.

"Permanent Gastrostomy As a Solution to Some Nutritional Problems in the Elderly," by Mark Pomerantz, Jacob Salomon, and Robert Dunn. *Journal of the American Geriatrics Society,* March 1980:104-107.

"The Patient Experiencing a Body Image Disturbance." *NCP Guide #2:29,* 2nd Ed., Nurseco, 1980.

"Tube Feedings: General Principles." *NCP Guide #5:50,* Nurseco, 1981.

The Patient with Glaucoma: Medical Treatment

Definition: Glaucoma is a disease characterized by increased tension or pressure within the eye and progressive loss of visual field.

LONG TERM GOAL: The patient will experience maximum therapeutic effect from compliance with medical regimen; the patient will adjust to limitations imposed by partial loss of vision.

General Considerations:
- **Incidence:** occurs in individuals past 40; second most common cause of blindness in US. An estimated 1 million Americans have undiagnosed glaucoma.
- Intraocular pressure increases as patient exerts energy (sneezing, running, bending over) or becomes emotionally upset; may also increase from excessive fluid intake or from use of certain medications (antihistamines or sympathomimetics).
- **Types and symptoms:** classified as primary or secondary. *Primary:* 1) chronic, simple, open-angle type occurs in 2% of population over 40; symptoms are insidious and develop slowly: mild discomfort, tired eye, impairment of peripheral vision, halos around lights; 2) congestive, closed-angle type is an *emergency* situation that may lead to blindness if left untreated; pressure increases rapidly with severe pain in and around eye, halos around lights, and blurred vision; may have nausea and vomiting. *Secondary:* many types secondary to conditions such as trauma, iritis, tumor, hemorrhage.
- **Prognosis:** the disease cannot be cured but can be controlled by treatment; early detection can reduce incidence of blindness.
- **Treatment** is aimed at controlling progress of disease with medication or surgery (see NCPG #5:10, "The Patient with Glaucoma: Surgical Treatment").
- **Nursing responsibilities** include teaching patient to adapt to medical regimen, counseling patient to adjust to limitations imposed by partial loss of vision, and to have annual eye check-ups with tonometry (measurement of eye pressure).

Specific Considerations, Potential Patient Outcomes, and Nursing Actions:

1) Drug Therapy

The patient verbalizes actions and side effects of prescribed medications, including symptoms to report to physician; patient demonstrates correct administration of eye medications:
- read physician's orders carefully for specific medications to each eye; the abbreviation for right eye is O.D., for left eye is O.L. *or* O.S., and for both eyes, O.U.;
- read labels carefully; accidental use of a *mydriatic agent can cause blindness in a person with glaucoma;* miotics constrict pupil & are used for glaucoma; see NCPG #5:44, "Drugs: Glaucoma;"

      — use sterile equipment & aseptic technique when administering medication to eye; place eyedrops carefully into everted lower lid; support your hand by placing finger on pt.'s forehead; do not allow eye dropper to touch eye or container of medication (may become a vehicle for spread of infection);

      — place ophthalmic ointment in a layer along inner surface of lower lid; instruct pt. to close eyes gently without squeezing them to help spread medication;

      — teach pt. to administer own eye medications; ensure that s/he can do it correctly.

2) Patient Education

The patient understands and complies with medical regimen; the patient demonstrates lifestyle changes to adjust to limitations imposed by partial loss of vision; the patient avoids activities that increase intraocular pressure:

— assess learning needs & anxiety level; health teach appropriate information as needed; see NCPG #1:49, "Teaching Patients: General Suggestions;"

— discuss any loss of vision that pt. has & adjustments that s/he will need to make for it;

— advise pt. to avoid activities that may increase intraocular pressure such as emotional upsets, intense excitement, exertion such as snow shoveling, pushing, or heavy lifting, constricting clothing such as tight girdles or belts, & upper respiratory infections;

— encourage maintenance of regular bowel habits with diet, fluids, & medications as ordered; straining on defecation causes increased intraocular pressure;

— plan daily moderate exercise; advise moderate use of eyes for reading, hobbies, & watching television;

— recommend wearing a medical identification tag indicating pt. has glaucoma;

— stress importance of continuous daily use of medications as prescribed & periodic checkups with ophthalmologist to keep condition under control;

— include family/significant others in teaching as necessary.

3) Psychosocial Adjustment

The patient expresses feelings and concerns about adjustment to partial loss of vision; the patient uses problem solving to increase ability to cope with stress and limitations of partial loss of vision:

— discuss & clarify beliefs, attitudes, & information about living with glaucoma with pt. & family;

— explore common pt. fears & concerns of blindness, threat to loss of independence, & frustration with limitations imposed by glaucoma; refer to NCPG #2:29,"The Patient Experiencing a Body Image Disturbance;"

— identify stressors in pt.'s daily life; problem solve to decrease stress & avoid emotional upsets; refer to NCPG #5:47."Problem Solving;"

— discuss any loss of vision that pt. has & adjustments that s/he will need to make for it;
— explore ability to participate in activities of daily living (ADL) & help cope with & adjust to limitations imposed by glaucoma;
— discuss new & alternative methods of dealing with stress; encourage moderate physical exercise that pt. enjoys to promote physical relaxation & emotional well being; refer to NCPG #5:49,"Stress Management;"
— if surgery is indicated, explore pt.'s feelings about proposed surgery, knowledge of possible outcome, family & work arrangements; support realistic problem solving & continued discussion amoung pt./family/friends.

Discharge Planning and Teaching Objectives/Outcomes

1) (Patient/Family/Significant Other) Can explain in own words basic facts about glaucoma, including nature of disease, symptoms, and medical maintenance regimen to control glaucoma.
2) Can state purpose, action, side effects of prescribed medications and can demonstrate correct administration of them.
3) Has been given written instructions re: exercise, medications, precautions, appointments with physician.
4) Has received information re: community resources for information and support.
5) Can state activities that may increase intraocular pressure and should be avoided, including excessive fluid intake, and use of antihistamines or sympathomimetic medications without medical management.
6) Has been advised to carry card or wear "dog tag" indicating individual has glaucoma.

Recommended References

"Drugs: Glaucoma." *NCP Guide #5:44.* Nurseco. 1981.
"Glaucoma: Diagnosis & Management" by D. Paton and J.A. Craig. *Clinical Symposia* 28-29. 1976:3-47.
"The Patient Experiencing a Body Image Disturbance." *NCP Guide #2:29.* 2nd Ed., Nurseco. 1980.
"The Patient with Glaucoma: Surgical Treatment." *NCP Guide #5:10.* Nurseco. 1981.
"Problem Solving." *NCP Guide #5:47.* Nurseco. 1981.
"Screening for Glaucoma." by Heather Boyd-Monk. *Nursing 79.* August 1979:42-45.
"Stress Management." *NCP Guide #5:49.* Nurseco. 1981.
"Teaching Patients: General Suggestions." *NCP Guide #1:49.* 2nd Ed., Nurseco. 1980.

The Patient with Glaucoma: Surgical Treatment

Definition: **Iridectomy** is an incision through the cornea so that a piece of the iris may be removed to facilitate drainage and thus reduce intraocular tension. Types are: *peripheral iridectomy* with small piece of iris removed at periphery, and *total or keyhole iridectomy* with larger piece of iris removed. *Irridencleisis* is an opening created between anterior chamber and the space beneath the conjunctiva so that aqueous fluid is absorbed into conjunctival tissues. *Trephination* is removal of a button of cornea and sclera to allow aqueous fluid to seep under the conjunction.

LONG TERM GOAL: The patient will recover from eye surgery for glaucoma without complications; the patient will return to usual roles in home, family, community after convalescence and will follow prescribed medical regimen.

General Considerations:

— **Indications:** surgery is done when glaucoma cannot be controlled medically; emergency surgery may be indicated for closed-angle glaucoma to halt rising intraocular pressure and to prevent optic nerve damage.

— **Treatment goal** of surgery is to produce an increased filtering channel so that there is more efficient outflow of aqueous fluid.

— **Nursing responsibilities include:** *pre-operatively,* 1) orienting patient to surroundings so that enviroment will be familiar to him when eye is covered; 2) teaching patient to breathe deeply and to do range of motion exercises (see NCPG #1:47) *without moving head;* 3) arranging for pre-operative measures as ordered by Dr.; 4) exploring fears and concerns, allowing and encouraging patient to express feelings; 5) if surgery is an emergency and time is short, staying with patient and family to relieve anxiety and fear, to explain procedures, and to answer questions (refer to NCPG #2:44, "General Preoperative Care"); *postoperatively,* monitoring the patient for prevention of complications, anxiety and fear, administering medications as ordered (refer to NCPGs #2:41, 42, 43, "General Postoperative Care").

Specific Considerations, Potential Patient Outcomes, and Nursing Actions:

1) Anxiety and Fear The patient/family experiences relief of fears and anxiety:

— be aware that surgery to the eye evokes fear of loss of vision; be attentive listener to pt./family concerns & feelings; know that providing information is one way to decrease anxiety;

— stay with pt. as much as possible; allow family/friend to stay quietly at bedside if pt. desires;

— announce yourself when you enter room; explain procedures & maintain a quiet, restful environment; reorient pt. to surroundings PRN;

    — administer analgesics as needed; do not make pt. wait for medication;

    — keep siderails up & leave call light so that pt. can reach it; place belongings closest to uninvolved eye so pt. can see them with minimal head movement;

    — refer to NCPGs #1:22, "The Patient Experiencing Anxiety," #1:28, "The Patient Experiencing Fear," & #1:32, "The Patient Experiencing Sensory Disturbances."

2) Prevention of Complications The patient recovers from glaucoma surgery free of preventable complications:

    — know that possible complications include: infection, increase in intraocular pressure, hemorrhage, injury to the eye; monitor pt. for early signs & symptoms of any of these;

    — position pt. as ordered (usually on back & on unoperated side, flat or with head of bed elevated);

    — instruct pt. to avoid activities that place stress on suture line, cause injury to eye or increase intraocular pressure such as rubbing eyes, brushing teeth or hair, bending over, moving quickly, sneezing, coughing;

    — notify physician immediately if pt. states there is sudden pain in eye; this may indicate hemorrhage;

    — give antiemetic drugs as ordered; provide cold compresses to throat for nausea & vomiting; stay with pt. & support head if vomiting; offer ice chips & liquid diet as ordered & tolerated;

    — guide pt. in deep breathing & range of motion exercises (to prevent complications of immobility) *without moving head;*

    — assist pt. to ambulate to bathroom when ordered; teach pt. to increase activities gradually (activity usually increased after initial dressing change by surgeon):

    — refer to NCPGs #2:41, 42, & 43, "General Postoperative Care."

3) Dressing The eye heals without infection, trauma, or bleeding; the eye dressing remains intact until surgeon changes it:

    — clarify eye dressing procedure with surgeon; initial dressing change will be done by surgeon; use strict aseptic technique & sterile equipment;

    — use eye shield to protect eye from injury;

    — report unusual drainage to surgeon immediately;

4) Drug Therapy Refer to NCPG #5:09, "The Patient with Glaucoma: Medical Treatment;" and #5:44, "Drugs: Glaucoma."

Discharge Planning and Teaching Objectives/Outcomes

1) (Patient/Family/Significant Other) Has written appointment date and time for follow-up care with surgeon; knows to report to surgeon any signs of infection or pain.
2) Can demonstrate correct eye dressing and medication procedures; can state dosage, frequency, actions, and side effects of medications.
3) Can state prescribed exercise and rest regimen, and activities to avoid.
4) Has received appropriate community referral to visiting nurse association or other community services.
5) Has been notified of continued need for periodic eye examinations by ophthalmologist.
6) Has been advised to carry card or "dog tag" indicating individual has glaucoma.

Recommended References

"Drugs: Glaucoma." *NCP Guide #5:44,* Nurseco, 1981.
"General Postoperative Care." *NCP Guides #2:41, 42, 43,* 2nd Ed., Nurseco, 1980.
"General Preoperative Care." *NCP Guide #2:44,* 2nd Ed., Nurseco, 1980.
"Glaucoma: Diagnosis and Management," by D. Paton and J.A. Craig. *Clinical Symposia,* 28-2, 1976:3-47.
"The Patient Experiencing Anxiety." *NCP Guide #1:22,* 2nd Ed., Nurseco, 1980.
"The Patient Experiencing Fear." *NCP Guide #1:28,* 2nd Ed., Nurseco, 1980.
"The Patient Experiencing Sensory Disturbances." *NCP Guide #1:32,* 2nd Ed., Nurseco, 1980.
"The Patient with Glaucoma: Medical Treatment." *NCP Guide #5:09,* Nurseco, 1981.
"Range of Motion Exercises." *NCP Guide #1:47,* 2nd Ed., Nurseco, 1980.

The Patient with Hodgkin's Disease

Definition: Hodgkin's Disease is a malignant lymphoma that chiefly affects the lymphatic structures (lymph nodes, spleen, thymus, Waldeyer's ring appendix, and Peyer's patches).

LONG TERM GOAL: The patient will experience maximum therapeutic effect from treatment plan; the patient and family will receive emotional support and adjust to limitations imposed by potential terminal illness.

General Considerations:
- **Incidence:** Hodgkin's Disease is a disease of the young and usually occurs between the ages of 20 to 40; there is a second rise in incidence from 55 to 75 years; males are affected more often than females.
- **Prognosis:** Over the last 20 years there has been a significant improvement in survival rates; an estimated 1 in 4 may live for 25 years with early treatment with radiation.
- **Cause** of the disease is unknown. The proliferating cells in Hodgkin's Disease are called Reed-Sternberg cells, a category of reticuloendothelial cell.
- **Typical progression:** the disease affects one lymph node and then travels through the lymphatic system to other lymph nodes or lymphatic structures of the body. The neoplastic process may extend to other organs and structures, liver, vertebrae, and to structures close to the involved lymphatic structures, e.g., ureters and bronchi. Progression of the disease may be fast or slow.
- **Stages of the Disease:**
  1) Involvement of one lymph node;
  2) Two or more lymph nodes involved on same side of diaphragm; or localized involvement of an organ plus one or more lymph node regions on same side of the diaphragm;
  3) Involvement of organs and tissues with or without lymph node involvement; and
  4) Involvement of skin, gastrointestional tract, liver, or bone marrow involvement away from the site of the involved lymph node(s).
- **Signs and symptoms:** The first symptom is a painless enlargement of lymph nodes, spleen, and liver, caused by the over-production of Reed-Sternberg cells. Severe pruritis is frequently present. Other early symptoms include fatigue, anorexia, irregular fever, increased susceptibility to infection. Later symptoms occur as the disease spreads and depend on the body structures/organs affected; they may include enlargement of the spleen and liver, jaundice, anemia, cough, dyspnea, chest pain, pleural effusion, pain in bones, compression of vertebrae, fracture (if disease disseminates to bones), pain in nerves and paralysis (if there is pressure on nerves or spinal cord). Continuous high fevers may indicate that death is near.

- **Diagnostic measures:** A laparotomy may be done to aid diagnosis. After the midline abdominal incision is made, affected nodes in the region are marked with clips that show up on x-ray; this helps keep account of the spread of the disease; splenectomy may be done, also to aid diagnosis (it is controversial as to whether it alters the cause of the disease or not); biopsies are taken of liver, ovaries, and lymph nodes.
- **Treatment** is aimed at eliminating the Reed-Sternberg cells from the body, protecting the patient from infection, and controlling symptoms to promote patient comfort:
  - Stages 1 & 2: Wide-field megavoltage radiation is given over a 4 to 6 week period. Often it is successful at eradicating the disease if not spread past lymph node chains, spleen, and nasopharynx.
  - Stages 3 & 4: Combined radiation and chemotherapy program. Drugs are usually given on a pattern of six courses, with 14 days on medication and 14 days off for rest and recuperation of bone marrow function in each course. See NCPG #5:48, "Radiation Therapy: General Principles."
  - Surgery is often initiated to provide relief from symptoms caused by pressure from a tumor mass, if the tumor can be removed.
  - Blood transfusions help control anemia.
  - Reverse isolation techniques protect against infections.
  - Emotional support is given to help the patient and family deal with the diagnosis of cancer, the noxious symptoms of both disease and treatments, and in the event that the disease progresses, to deal with the patient's approaching death.
- **Nursing responsibilities** include alleviating the patient's symptoms to maintain optimal comfort and nutrition, observing and reporting signs and symptoms, maintaining strict reverse isolation to protect the patient from infection, and ministering to the patient's and family's needs for emotional care.

Specific Considerations, Potential Patient Outcomes, and Nursing Actions:

1) Knowledge of Disease

Patient/Family/Significant Other (SO) know the effects of Hodgkin's Disease on the body, the treatment modalities, positive chance for cure, the control of treatment complications, the importance of early detection and treatment of recurrences:
  - teach pt. the typical course of the disease: explain symptoms for the stage that pt. is experiencing; teach that the course of the disease & treatment are long-term;
  - explain treatments: radiation for localized tumor destruction, chemotherapy for systemic treatment; inform pt. of the side effects of the therapy prescribed; see NCPG #4:44, "Drugs: Antileukemic;"

2) Prevention of Infection

Patient remains free of hospital-based infections and remains in an infection-free state:
— explain to pt. that his disease and treatment lower his resistance & make him prone to infections; instruct on general health-prevention measures, e.g., hand washing, a diet high in protein, iron & vitamins, adequate rest, & avoidance of infectious persons;
— keep pt. away from infectious persons (pts., staff, visitors); wash your hands before beginning to care for pt. (giving medications, treatments, or other procedures);
— monitor vital signs; be aware of increases in TPR as indicators of infections & report to physician immediately.

3) Control of Symptoms

Patient has side effects of disease and treatment monitored and treated; patient is as free of noxious stimuli as possible:
— assess for pain of abdomen, bones, chest and other areas caused by disease process Q2-3H when awake; medicate as ordered:
— provide sedation at night if needed; offer backrubs, pillows, relaxation tapes, & other comfort measures;
— know that anticipatory nausea & vomiting before chemotherapy is common; medicate pt. when it happens; administer antiemetics before, during, & after chemotherapy PRN;
— monitor & chart pt.'s responses to chemotherapy, antiemetics, sedatives; communicate closely with the physician;
— know that fatigue & depression accompany the treatment of the disease; encourage pt. to talk about his fears & feelings; be an attentive listener;
— provide bulk in the diet, e.g., bran & fresh vegetables, to prevent constipation; a stool softener is effective for constipation; for diarrhea, give yogurt, if tolerated, to restock depleted lactobacilli supply;
— for dry cough after radiation, use humidifier, lozenges to reduce dry tickle;
— be aware of chemotherapy agents the pt. is receiving; know & watch for side effects that are usual (e.g., nausea, anemia, alopecia) & side effects that indicate a potential danger to the pt. (e.g., leukopenia, thrombocytopenia, bone marrow suppression); consult pharmacist, the physician, PDR, & pharmacology book PRN.

4) Psychosocial Adjustment

Patient recognizes own level of activity, that symptoms will persist, and that length of treatment and disease may last for years; patient incorporates these facts into own activities of daily living and relationships with others; patient describes plan for living in the present:

— encourage pt. to discuss feelings & fears for the present & the future; inform pt. that many hospitalizations in the future are probable;

— discuss with pt. & family the importance of living in the present; the disease process & treatment are lengthy & exacerbations are to be expected; the future is uncertain;

— explore with pt. & family what pt. is capable of engaging in today; encourage the emphasis of living for each day;

— be aware that some days pt. will feel better than others; activities of the day can be planned according to pt.'s energy level;

— have pt. consider & discuss what activities will be engaged in after discharge & what activities will be discontinued;

— encourage pt. to continue work, either outside the home or at home as tolerated: i.e., 3-4 hours a day, since work gives a person a sense of purpose, accomplishment, identity, & self-worth;

— encourage continuance of friendships as tolerated; include family & SO in planning as much as possible; offer emotional support & encourage family/SO to discuss concerns & feelings;

— assess for depression; have pt. verbalize feelings; refer to NCPG #1:26, "The Patient Experiencing Depression;" discuss referral to a psychotherapist with pt.;

— discuss with pt. the changed body image; have pt. talk about its effect on life & relationships; consult NCPG #2:29, "The Patient Experiencing a Body Image Disturbance;"

— discuss positive aspects: activities pt. can do, support from family/friends, strengths, positive coping mechanisms;

— inform pt. of support groups available, e.g., the American Cancer Society, Make Today Count, church groups, volunteer organizations;

— refer to NCPGs #1:27, "Dealing with Impending Death," & #1:31, "Responses to Loss," when warranted by pt.'s condition; also see NCPG #5:45, "Hospice Care Concepts."

Discharge Planning and Teaching Objectives/Outcomes
1) (Patient/Family/Significant Other) Has an appointment with physician for follow-up care.

2) Knows to call doctor immediately for signs of enlarged glands, pain, elevated TPR, or other signs of infection.
3) Knows action and side effects of medication to be taken for control of symptoms: pain medication, antiemetic, stool softeners, cough, and others depending on symptoms exhibited.
4) Knows to call physician immediately if s/he experiences dangerous side effects of chemotherapy agents.
5) Knows fatigue, depression, cough, weight loss will last up to one year after treatment stops; has a plan to cope with these symptoms.
6) Knows of support groups in home area and the name and phone number of the contact person.

Recommended References

"Dealing with Impending Death." *NCP Guide #1:27*, 2nd Ed., Nurseco, 1980.

"Drugs: Antileukemin." *NCP Guide #4:44*, Nurseco, 1978.

"Hodgkin Disease. A Nursing Care Study, with the Patient's Own Side of the Story," by A. Harwood. *Nursing Times*, Sept. 20, 1979:1617-1623.

"Hospice Care Concepts." *NCP Guide #5:45*, Nurseco, 1981.

"The Patient Experiencing a Body Image Disturbance." *NCP Guide #2:29*, 2nd Ed., Nurseco, 1980.

"The Patient Experiencing Depression." *NCP Guide #1:26*, 2nd. Ed., Nurseco, 1980.

"People with Hodgkin Disease: The Nursing Challenge," by D. H. LeBlanc. *Nursing Clinics of North America*, June 1978:281-300.

"Radiation Therapy: General Principles." *NCP Guide #5:48*, Nurseco, 1981.

"Responses to Loss: The Grief and Mourning Process." *NCP Guide #1:31*, 2nd Ed., Nurseco, 1980.

"Working Towards a Cure for All," by I. E. Smith. *Nursing Mirror*, December 7, 1978:37-39.

The Patient with Infectious Mononucleosis

Definition: Infectious Mononucleosis is an acute infectious disease of the lymphatic system caused by the Epstein-Barr virus, a DNA virus of the herpes-virus group.

LONG TERM GOAL: The patient will recover from acute phase free of preventable complications, and will adhere to prescribed medical regimen planned to prevent complications until recovery is complete.

General Considerations:
- **Etiology:** transmission of mononucleosis is by oral contact; the virus may persist in the pharynx for weeks or months, so carriers are common in the convalescent period. The virus can also be spread by blood transfusion. Incubation period is from 30 to 50 days.
- Immunity occurs if a primary infection with Epstein-Barr virus (EBV) develops in childhood, causing a mild and nonspecific or inapparent illness with resulting antibody to EBV. If an individual without antibody to EBV acquires the infection, clinical manifestations of mononucleosis occur in approximately 50% of the cases; the 15-25 year old population is most commonly affected.
- **Symptoms** include fever, sore throat, fatigue, lethargy, headache, lymph node enlargement, and supraorbital edema. Enlarged spleen, hepatitis, and secondary infection are common complications.
- **Diagnosis** can be made from clinical symptoms and laboratory findings of abnormal lymphocytes, a positive heterophil-antibody test, abnormal liver-function tests.
- **Treatment** is symptomatic and supportive; most patients recover in 1 to 3 weeks, with aspirin for fever, headache, and muscle pains and bedrest while fever continues. Steroids may be given for complications of hepatic dysfunction, neurological symptoms, or severe symptoms or thrombocytopenia, hemolytic anemia, or airway obstruction. Isolation precautions are not necessary after diagnosis is confirmed; patient should be informed of carrier status and taught to avoid oral contact for 2 months.
- **Nursing responsibilities** include assessing for symptoms and complications, prescribing nursing interventions, providing drug therapy as ordered, and teaching patient/family/significant other (SO) measures to help prevent complications and spread of disease.

Specific Considerations, Potential Patient Outcomes, and Nursing Actions:
1) Fever and Hydration   The patient regains a normal body temperature; the patient maintains a normal fluid balance:
   - check vital signs at least Q4H & PRN; provide cooling measures (sponges, etc.) for temperature over 102; give

aspirin for fever as ordered;
- check linens for dampness from perspiration & change PRN; prevent pt. from chilling;
- monitor skin, tongue, I&O for signs of dehydration; refer to NCPGs #3:48 & 49, "Fluids and Electrolytes, Parts A and B;"
- offer bland fluids frequently; if pt. has anorexia or sore throat, offer 6 small, soft meals; check with pt. for preference of warm or cool food/fluids, likes & dislikes.

2) Rest, Comfort, and Exercise

The patient maintains an adequate rest pattern; the patient is free of fever, sore throat, headache, and muscle pains; the patient experiences increased comfort and alternates periods of rest and activity:
- encourage pt. to remain on bedrest as long as fever persists; explain to pt. that the body must rest to prevent complications; while pt. is on bedrest, provide active ROM excercises at least TID (see NCPG #1:47);
- be aware that relationships with peers & acceptance of peers are issues of great importance to the adolescent & young adult; developmental behaviors of rebellion & severe criticism of authority may also be present; spend time listening to pt.'s feelings, concerns, & preferences, & utilize these in planning care; know that unless the young person is involved in planning care, issues of rebellion & non-compliance to treatment plan will be a problem; see NCPGs #3:26, "Normal Growth & Development: The Adolescent" & #5:33 "The Patient Manifesting Non-Compliance;"
- assess for sore throat, headache, & muscle pain Q4H during waking hours; offer analgesics as ordered; give backrubs & comfort measures;
- plan care around rest periods; assess pt. for favorite ways to relax & assist pt. to problem solve to adapt to limitations due to sick role; examples: pt. may use earphones to listen to music, relaxation tapes, or radio, listen to a friend read, watch television, observe birds or a fishtank, play quiet games such as cards, do crossword puzzles, stitchery, or art work; projects that can be worked at for a short time & set aside during rest periods work best; see NCPGs #5:47, "Problem Solving" & #5:36, "The Patient Adapting to The Sick Role."
- know that pt. may have fatigue & low energy for weeks & months after acute symptoms subside; explain to pt./family/SO the importance of daily rest periods to promote healing;

3) Prevention of Complications

The patient is free of preventable complications; the patient/family/SO describes life style changes to prevent complications and promote healing:

- know that the enlarged spleen is vulnerable to injury & may rupture if subjected to even mild trauma; symtoms of rupture of the spleen include abdominal pain & shoulder pain from the presence of free intraperitoneal blood irritating the diaphragm; these symptoms should be reported to physician immediately; treatment includes blood transfusions & immediate splenectomy:
- advise pt. to avoid rough-housing, strenuous physical activity, & competitive sports until recovery is complete; this may be a period of 2-6 months & should be determined by physician;
- observe for symptoms of marked hepatic dysfunction during acute phase of illness; these may include persistent fever, neurological manifestations, thrombocytopenia, hemolytic anemia, airway obstruction, jaundice, continued presence of anorexia, & abnormal liver-function tests; report these symptoms to physician; steroids may be used when severe or life-threatening complications develop;
- know that pt. is susceptible to secondary infection; use good hand washing technique; exposure to visitors during the first week or two of acute symptoms should be kept to a minimum; teach pt./family/SO the importance of good hygiene measures to prevent secondary infection while resistance is down;
- problem solve with pt./family/SO to determine a realistic schedule to return to usual social life & activities; instruct the pt. to listen to messages from body to determine fatigue level, & to plan to alternate short periods of activity with rest periods for 2-3 months; know that this limitation may be very frustrating to young person; give emotional support by listening to feelings & attitude toward creative problem solving;
- instruct pt. to avoid immunizations for about 6 months after symptoms subside (cellular immune reactivity remains reduced for some time).

Discharge Planning and Teaching Objectives/Outcomes

1) (Patient/Family/Significant Other) Knows implications of carrier status and agrees to avoid oral contact for 2 months; can describe hygiene measures and plan for adequate rest and nutrition to prevent secondary infection while resistance is reduced.
2) Can describe symptoms of secondary infection, marked hepatic dysfunction, and ruptured spleen; knows to call physician immediately if these symptoms occur.
3) Can describe plan to avoid strenuous physical activity and competitive sports until physician states recovery is complete.

Recommended References

"Fluids & Electrolytes, Parts A & B." *NCP Guides #3:48, 49,* Nurseco, 1977.

"Infectious Mononucleosis," by F. Shurin. *Pediatric Clinics of North America,* May 1979:315.

"Normal Growth & Development: The Adolescent." *NCP Guide #3:26,* Nurseco, 1977.

"The Patient Adapting to the Sick Role." *NCP Guide #5:36,* Nurseco, 1981.

"The Patient Manifesting Non-Compliance." *NCP Guide #5:33,* Nurseco, 1981.

"Problem Solving." *NCP Guide #5:47,* Nurseco, 1981.

"Range of Motion Exercises." *NCP Guide #1:47,* 2nd Ed., Nurseco, 1980.

The Patient who is Obese

Definition: Obesity is most often defined as the state of being more than 20 percent overweight for height and build standards of ideal body weight (IBW).

LONG TERM GOAL: The obese patient will experience sensitive acceptance and alert concern for welfare while hospitalized or attending out-patient clinics; the obese patient will be assisted to accept and adjust to a comprehensive program of weight management.

General Considerations:

— **Risk:** Overweight persons (5-20% over IBW), seem to carry some increased risk to health, but must be evaluated on an individual basis as to need for a serious program of weight management. Of greater immediate concern are those individuals who are more than 20% above their IBW. Hypertension, myocardial infarction, strokes, and other cardiovascular disease are commonly associated with obesity. There is also a greater incidence of diabetes mellitus, gallstones, and gynecological disorders.

The hospitalized and bedfast obese patient has a much more difficult recovery from medical or surgical conditions. Postoperative wound healing is complicated by increased likelihood of dehiscence and infection. Difficulty moving the obese bed patient heightens the possibilities for atelectasis, pneumonia, hypoventilation, emboli, and thrombophlebitis. Increased demand on the heart contributes to possible dysrhythmias, pulmonary edema, and circulatory overload. There are more secondary complications involving renal, hepatic, integumentary, and endocrine systems than for a normal weight person.

— **Pickwickian Syndrome,** also called obesity hypoventilation, is common in the severely obese of both sexes, all ages. Characteristics involve frequent periods of nighttime apnea (15-90 sec.) causing restless sleep disturbance and daytime somnolence. Respiratory stimulant medications that seem to work include progesterone and tricyclic antidepressants. Significant weight reduction is the treatment of choice.

— **Diagnostic assessment** includes history of onset of overweight, distribution of body fat, abnormal metabolic findings (glucose tolerance, serum cholesterol, triglyceride levels, hypertension, etc.), patterns of eating and activity, psychosocial factors and family/friend support systems, complete physical exam, chest x-rays, electrocardiogram, and endocrine studies when indicated.

— **Treatment Program:** To achieve a goal of reaching and maintaining ideal body weight while still maintaining health, treatment must include:
(1) patient/family education and counseling for attitude and behavior change;
(2) diet to lower caloric intake yet provide balanced nutrients;
(3) activity increase to expend more calories; and

(4) continuing medical, nutritional, and psychological supervision and support

Unsatisfactory weight-loss therapies with temporary or limited success and undesirable side effects or complications include pills (amphetamines and other appetite depressants, diuretics, human chorionic gonadotropin), acupuncture, massage/vibration machines, jaw wiring, fasting, bypass surgery, and liquid protein, ketogenic, or fad diets. Because these do not usually involve permanent attitude and behavior changes, weight losses are not likely to be maintained.

Gaining in popularity and success are treatments which involve behavior modification, hypnosis, imagery, conditioning, enviromental management, contingency management, support groups, exercise programs (aerobic dancing, slim and trim classes, jogging, swimming, walking), and nutritionally balanced, low-caloric diets (that fit client's food preferences and life style).

- **Nursing responsibilities** include:
    (1) assisting with assessment of individual's health and nutrition status;
    (2) assisting patient with problem identification, goal setting, and problem-solving plan;
    (3) planning, implementing, and evaluating care modified to meet needs of obese patient;
    (4) interpreting dietary prescription and providing nutrition education PRN; and
    (5) making appropriate referrals to nutrition specialist, psychological counselor, group therapy program, and/or published sources of reliable nutrition and weight loss information.

- **Diet Clubs:** mutual support, peer-related, self-help groups are often valuable to sustaining interest and commitment to a long-range program of weight reduction. It is important that the group chosen has a philosophy and approach that is acceptable to patient as well as a membership with whom s/he can readily identify. Those most successful are often job-related, age-relevant or sex, and socio-economic group-based. The group's goals include mutual honesty and acceptance, willingness to listen and help others, growth in confidence, self-understanding and self-esteem, and continuing encouragement to achieve and maintain personal weight reduction goal.

Compulsive overeaters have found help with a group known nationally as Overeaters Anonymous, patterned after Alcoholics Anonymous. Further information can be obtained from: Overeaters Anonymous World Service Office, 2190 -190th St., Torrance, CA 90504, or see white pages of local telephone directory. A similar non-profit diet organization is TOPS (Take Off Pounds Sensibly), PO Box 07489, Milwaukee, WI 53207. Perhaps most well-known is Weight Watchers International, Inc., 800 Community Drive, Manhasset, NY 11030. Diet/exercise/counseling and behavior modification groups can also be found in local medical centers and hospitals, health maintenance organizations, schools and colleges as well as many businesses.

Specific Considerations, Potential Patient Outcomes, and Nursing Actions:

1) Hospitali-
   zation

The hospitalized patient receives intensive care modified to prevent complications associated with obesity; the hospitalized patient experiences acceptance by staff who willingly accommodate changes necessitated by the patient's size:

- adapt bed by using extra firm mattress over a bed board; set up overhead frame with trapeze to assist moving pt.; for the patient over 400 lbs., wire two bedframes together & place two mattresses sideways;
- if necessary, weigh pt. by placing two standing scales side by side & adding sum of two readings; for the pt. over 400 lbs., take pt. to hospital's freight scale;
- turn pt. using long, strong regular sheets folded as pull sheets; plan on having extra persons to help lift pt. so that embarrassment can be avoided; use a Hoyer lift if needed to get pt. up; over 400 lbs., rent or borrow a Transaide lift;
- ask engineering to construct a wider walker using bed frame parts; ask family to bring in own sitting chair or made-to-order wheelchair;
- be especially observant for cardiopulmonary complications of hypoxemia, cyanosis, hypercapnia; know & report abnormal CO_2 & PAO_2 levels; keep emergency equipment accessible & ready for use; turn, cough & deep breathe pt. Q2H; provide range of motion exercises at least Q4H (see NCPG #1:47);
- check BP before & after getting pt. out of bed; observe safety precautions to prevent falls associated with postural hypotension & dizziness;
- notify other depts. in advance of pt.'s visit so that preparations & accommodations can be made;
- supervise skin care to ascertain that skin is kept clean, dry, & free of irritation; use powder & cotton fabric or padding between skin folds; use antiperspirants & deodorants; check room for adequacy of ventilation;
- use longer needles for injections: IM length for SC medications, & spinal length needles for IM injections; get the most skilled therapist to start IVs & take precautions to protect venipuncture site from trauma;
- encourage pt. to wear own nightwear or ask linen room staff to sew a special gown for pt.;
- observe & report periods of nighttime apnea & restless sleep disturbance as well as daytime somnolence; change pt.'s position to semi-Fowler's or prone; give prescribed medications that may be helpful for stimulating respiration.

2) Diet

The patient's IBW is determined and a dietary prescription is calculated; the patient states own energy and nutrient requirements; the patient describes and develops dailyl and weekly diet plans appropriate to own life style requirements; the patient achieves IBW with sufficient balanced nutrients for wellness:
- consult with physician, dietician, pt./family/friends to develop an individualized, suitable dietary prescription;
- interpret diet to pt./family/friends; encourage questions & invite participation in planning menus, cooking adaptations, dining out policies;
- teach pt./family/friends "general rules" for sensible dieting; refer to NCPG #5:41, "Diet: Weight Control;"
- weigh pt. & provide record ro pt. to keep; give appt. for follow-up visits to doctor's office or weight control clinic;
- provide written food lists, instruction, & reliable nutrition references for pt. to take home.

3) Exercise

The patient helps to plan own exercise program; the patient participates regularly in selected exercise mode:
- study (or take yourself) history to learn what physical activities are done by pt.. for how long & how often; find out what activities have been tried & rejected by pt. & why; learn what activities are encouraged by family or friends & what activities are most likely to be acceptable to pt.;
- assess knowledge & misconceptions of pt./family re: exercise/activity & health teach PRN (for example, many think that exercise increases appetite, but the opposite is true for the overweight person);
- consider walking as the most practical. cheapest, easiest, most acceptable, & tolerated activity; increase time & distance weekly to six miles;
- discuss exercise regimen with pt.'s physician to ensure that program is medically safe for pt.;
- refer to physical therapist for a planned program of exercise, if necessary.

4) Psychosocial Adjustment

The patient experiences interest, support, and acceptance by staff and family/friends; the patient has a positive attitude about self and weight management program:
- become acquainted with the pt.'s obesity history, patterns of weight gain & loss, & psychosocial problems; be careful of pt.'s feelings, avoiding embarrassment or resentment by providing privacy & using tact when asking questions;
- encourage pt. to express feelings & tell you about self & attitudes toward previous weight loss efforts; try to determine if pt. feels obese condition is reversible or has given up; remember the ultimate decision to embark

on another weight management program rests with pt.; try to instill hope for change but refrain from lecturing, shaming, or giving unwanted advice;

— know that motivation has to come from within pt.; learn what reasons pt. has for wanting to lose weight, what desire for change was present in past efforts, what motivation (external or internal) the pt. thinks is needed for success this time;

— use various strategies to increase pt.'s self-esteem & to accept a new, slimmer body image; try visual imagery techniques; refer to NCPGs #5:37, "Behavior Modification," #2:29, "The Patient Experiencing a Body Image Disturbance," & #5:32, "The Patient Experiencing a Threat to Self-Esteem;"

— help pt. to locate an appropriate mutual-support peer group or diet club within community with which s/he can identify; explore occupationally-related groups for working persons, neighborhood gym/spa or church-related groups for housewives, senior centers for older clients & teenage groups for adolescents;

— teach pt./family how to deal with dietary/weight loss "set-backs" often related to situational crises; see NCPG #5:31, "The Patient Experiencing Guilt;"

— teach pt./family to select rewards for goal achievement that are non-food oriented (psychosocial & physical pleasures & material gifts such as flowers, theater tickets, clothers, music tapes & records).

5) Behavior Modification

The patient identifies causes of weight problems; the patient develops and practices life style modifications of diet, exercise, and stress-coping techniques:

— teach pt. how to keep a food record or diary that includes: amount & type of food or drink consumed, with whom, when, location, type of activity or situation while eating, subjective feelings or mood, & level of hunger;

— help pt. identify own problem behaviors & set goals for self; refer to NCPG #5:42, "Problem Solving;"

— help pt. select strategies related to identified problem & set goal; provide pt. with information so that s/he can consider aversive conditioning (associating an unpleasant stimulus with a favorite food), contingency management (attaching consequences to desirable & undesirable eating behaviors), environmental management (seeking changes to reinforce positive behaviors), visual imagery (imagining self with new body image & attitude toward food), or hypnotic suggestion; see NCPG #5:37, "Behavior Modification;"

— help pt. to utilize strategies selected or refer to a competent psychologist, nurse practitioner, or counselor who can help.

Discharge Planning and Teaching Objectives/Outcomes

1) (Patient/Family/Significant Other) Can explain in own terms the relationship between obesity and chronic health problems.
2) Can identify which risk factors s/he has and can tell how s/he can modify them in own favor.
3) Can state own energy and nutrient requirements along with ideal body weight goal.
4) Can identify own causes of weight problems (e.g., rate, frequency, amount of eating; content of diet; emotional or social reasons) and how s/he will try to handle these.
5) Has developed own goals and personal intervention programs that includes desirable life style modifications of diet, exercise, and eating patterns.
6) Has developed plans for using assistance of group therapy, private counseling or diet club method; has written daily and weekly diet plans; has a contingency plan for a break in diet or set-back; has a plan to control eating in restaurants and other people's homes; and is able to accept alternative activities for uncontrolled eating.
7) Agrees to return regularly as appointed to weight control therapist (MD, RN, other professional); accepts idea that permanent weight reduction and control is a long-range program requiring continuing supervision and pschological support.

Recommended References

"A Sensible Approach to the Obese Patient," by L. Kathleen Mahan. *Nursing Clinics of North America,* June 1979:229-245.
"Behavior Modification." *NCP Guide #5:37*, Nurseco, 1981.
"Diet: Weight Control. *NCP Guide #5:41*, Nurseco, 1981.
"Solving the Very Big Problems of the Morbidly Obese," by Ginger Kawasaki et al. *Nursing 80,* November 1980:40-43
"Problem Solving." *NCP Guide #5:47*, Nurseco, 1981.
"The Patient Experiencing a Body Image Disturbance." *NCPG #2:29*, 2nd Ed., Nurseco, 1980.
"The Patient Experiencing Guilt." *NCPG #5:31*, Nurseco, 1981.
"The Patient Experiencing a Threat to Self-Esteem." *NCPG #5:32*, Nurseco, 1981.
"Range of Motion Exercises." *NCP Guide #1:47*, 2nd Ed., Nurseco, 1980.
"When Your Client Has A Weight Problem:
　Nursing Assessment," by Jane White and Mary Ann Schroeder.
　Nursing Management," by Mary L. Kornguth.
　Pickwickian Syndrome," by Carol McCreary and Juanita Watson.
　Teenagers and Obesity," by Rae Langford.
　Overeaters Anonymous: A Self-Help Group." *The American Journal of Nursing,* March 1981:549-564.

The Patient with Pelvic Radiation (External)

Definition: External radiation therapy is the treatment of a person with roentgen rays for the purpose of destroying malignant cells or to make them incapable of further cell division.

LONG TERM GOAL: The patient will experience maximum therapeutic benefit from radiation treatments, adjust to psychosocial implications of potential terminal illness that may or may not be cured, and return to family, home, occupation with minimal limitations and side effects.

General Considerations:
— **Indications** for external pelvic radiation are female/male carcinoma of the reproductive system, lower gastrointestinal system, or lower urinary system.
— Pelvic radiation may be performed as a primary, single modality, or as an adjunctive, synergistic therapy in treatment of cancer. Combination modalities may include pre- or postoperative external radiation or radioactive isotope implantation, surgery, immunotherapy, and/or chemotherapy.
— **Side effects** of external pelvic radiation therapy may include gastrointestinal disturbances, hematuria, frequency, a drop in blood count, and anemia. Refer to NCPG #5:48, "Radiation Therapy: General Principles," for further information.
— **Nursing responsibilities** include assisting the patient/family to accept/adapt to psychosocial and physical impact of cancer and its recommended treatment, intervening to minimize disagreeable and uncomfortable side effects of radiation therapy, encouraging skillful and self-confident independence as far as possible, participating in treatment and planning for discharge, and, referring patient to counseling, financial aid, home care, and physical or medical assistance.

Specific Considerations, Potential Patient Outcomes, and Nursing Actions:
1) Psychosocial Adjustment   The patient understands and accepts the objectives, implications, and potential side effects of pelvic radiation therapy with lessened fear, growing confidence and a positive, optimistic attitude:
   — assess pt./family knowledge of radiation treatment in relation to own disease process & expected therapy outcomes;
   — encourage pt. to express fears, anxieties, doubts, & misunderstandings; take time to actively listen to pt./family; promote a warm, concerned environment conducive to free exchange of feelings;

- explain to pt./family what they want & need to know re: treatment process & procedures, radiation effects, & what is expected of pt./family to support positive outcomes;
- encourage participation & independence in planning & giving care to foster pt.'s sense of personal control;
- promote some socialization, counseling, & communication opportunities for depressed or withdrawn pts; refer to NCPG #1:26, "The Patient Experiencing Depression;"

2) Radiation Syndrome (Sickness)

The patient understands and copes with predictable symptoms of radiation sickness; the patient participates in overcoming and minimizing complications and problems:
- observe & record skin dryness, redness, tautness & desquamation; cleanse gently only with approved solutions (usually only tepid water) & apply emollient ointments only as prescribed; explain to pt. temporary nature of these skin changes; keep linens next to skin soft, non-starched, non-binding;
- note & record GI reactions of nausea, vomiting, anorexia, diarrhea; administer sedatives, analgesics, antihistamines, antiemetics, & antidiarrheic medications PRN as ordered;
- monitor parenteral therapy; record I&O; encourage fluid intake when able to keep down oral fluids;
- consult with dietitian so individual preferences & needs may be considered;
- give vitamin & mineral supplements ordered;
- encourage family or friends to be present during meals, as encouragement & companionship help to stimulate appetite & increase amt. eaten;
- refer to NCPG #5:48, "Radiation Therapy: General Principles," for additional information on nutrition suggestions.

3) Adjunctive Therapy

The patient understands, adapts to and participates positively in concurrent medical/surgical treatments for cancer:
- refer to NCPG #2:07, "The Patient with Cancer: Early Stages;" see also NCPG #2:08, "The Patient with Cancer: Advanced Stages;"
- refer to NCPG #5:16, "The Patient with Radiation Implant/GYN," if this treatment method is used.

Discharge Planning and Teaching Objectives/Outcomes
1) (Patient/Family/Significant Other) Is aware of amount and kind of care patient will need at home, and has verbalized confidence in a realistic arrangement or plan to provide it.

2) Has been referred to a nursing home, convalescent hospital, or home health agency (VNA or private community nursing resource); has phone number and leaflet describing services of local American Cancer Society.
3) Knows that douches and enemas may relieve residual irritation and knows how to administer these with prescribed solution.
4) Knows to resume activities gradually over time as fatigue and lethargy subside and patient feels stronger; knows importance of balancing rest with passive and active exercises and can demonstrate these.
5) Knows to avoid direct sunlight on skin areas exposed to radiation as well as irritating soaps; has an emollient cream or lotion for relief of dryness or itching.
6) Knows to observe and report promptly to physician any frequency or burning urination, diarrhea, continuing nausea, vomiting or anorexia, temperature over 100°F., and any severe pain as well as redness, warmth and tenderness in venipuncture sites or legs.

Recommended References

"Fatigue in Patients Receiving Localized Radiation," by Pamela Haylock and Laura Hart. *Cancer Nursing*, December 1979:461-467.

"Nutritional Problems in Radiotherapy Patients," by James C. Rose. *The American Journal of Nursing*, July 1978:1194-1196.

"Radiation Therapy: General Principles." *NCP Guide #5:48*, Nurseco, 1981.

"The Patient Experiencing Depression." *NCP Guide #1:26*, 2nd Ed., Nurseco, 1980.

"The Patient with Cancer: Advanced Stages." *NCP Guide #2:08*, 2nd Ed., Nurseco, 1980.

"The Patient with Cancer: Early Stages." *NCP Guide #2:07*, 2nd Ed., Nurseco, 1980.

"The Patient with Radiation Implant/GYN." *NCP Guide #5:16*, Nurseco, 1981.

The Patient with Pernicious Anemia

Definition: Pernicious anemia is a chronic, progressive anemia of adults caused by a deficiency in secretion of the intrinsic factor by the gastric mucosa.

LONG TERM GOAL: The patient will continue prescribed vitamin B-12 injections and diet and adapt to limitations imposed by chronic disease.

General Considerations:
- **Etiology:** the intrinsic factor deficiency results in malabsorption of vitamin B-12 from the gastrointestinal tract. The vitamin B-12 deficiency diminishes DNA synthesis, resulting in defective maturation of cells of the bone marrow and gastrointestinal tract. The disease is treatable, but is fatal if not controlled.
- **Incidence:** occurs mainly in people of both sexes over 50 years old; fair-complexioned people are most susceptible.
- **Major characteristics** of the disease are abnormally large erythrocytes (macrocytosis); deficiency of hydrochloric acid in gastric juice (hypochlorhydria); neurological and gastrointestinal symptoms and fatal outcome without treatment. Lack of vitamin B-12 also affects peripheral nerves, spinal cord, and the brain; these symptoms are reduced with injections of vitamin B-12. Three quarters of the patients with pernicious anemia develop symptoms of central nervous systems dysfunction. Permanent neurologic damage occurs in extreme cases and is not helped by vitamin B-12 injections.
- **Causes:** heredity, prolonged iron deficiency, autoimmune disorder, total gastrectomy, and sometimes partial gastrectomy or gastrojejunostomy for peptic ulcer.
- **Signs and symptoms:** weakness, pallor, fatigue, dyspnea, palpitations, jaundice, sore mouth, smooth, beefy-red tongue, weight loss, indigestion, constipation, or diarrhea. Tingling, numbness in hands and feet, depression, and confusion are symptoms caused by neurologic impairment.
- **Diagnostic tests:**
  - Schilling test is the definitive test for pernicious anemia, as it tests for lack of the intrinsic factor.
  - Gastric juice analysis shows decreased free hydrochloric acid, high pH and low volume.
  - RBC: erthrocyte count below 3 million red blood cells/100ml; erythrocytes are oval and macrocytic.
  - Bone marrow aspiration contains high numbers of megaloblasts, few normablasts or normally maturing erythrocytes, and defects in maturation of leucocytes.
  - Unconjugated bilirubin elevated; serum LDH activity is extremely high.

— **Treatment:** patients need both immediate and life-long therapy consisting of:
  - Injections of vitamin B-12 for a lifetime.
  - Ferrous sulfate or ferrous gluconate (if hemoglobin level fails to rise in proportion to increase in erythrocyte count).
  - Blood transfusions are given in severe anemia.
  - Nutritious diet high in iron, protein, and vitamins.
  - Restricted activity, ranging from bedrest to alternating limited activity and frequent rest periods as dictated by severity of the anemia.
  - Protection from burns and other forms of trauma since patients have reduced sensations of heat and pain.
  - Folic acid is controversial as treatment.
  - Blood transfusions are given in severe anemia.

— **Nursing responsibilities** involve implementation of medical teaching plan, teaching the patient the cause and treatment of his disease, and helping him to adapt to the limitations of this chronic disease (see NCPG #5:30, "The Patient Adapting to Chronic Illness Role.")

Specific Considerations, Potential Patient Outcomes, and Nursing Actions:

1) Diet and Drug Therapy

The patient describes cause of illness and treatment plan; the patient establishes and maintains a schedule of vitamin B-12 injections; the patient ingests a nutritious diet high in iron, proteins and vitamins:
  - teach pt. & family/significant other (SO) the cause of the illness & how it can be controlled; be sure pt. understands cause & treatment;
  - ask dietician to explain to pt. & the one who prepares the pt.'s meals the importance of eating foods that are high in iron, vitamins, & protein; arrange to have these foods served to pt; provide printed materials that identify such foods;
  - assess dietary intake; communicate closely with doctor & dietician re: adequacy of intake; change menu offerings as necessary; smaller meals or snacks in the afternoon & before bedtime may be more palatable to pt. & help him to eat more food;
  - with dietician's aid, help pt. & the one who prepares pt.'s meals to devise a sample week's menu;
  - administer vitamin B-12 injections & other medications & treatments as ordered; explain rationale to pt.

2) Relief of   Patient has symptoms controlled and is as active and comfortable as possible:
   Symptoms
- assess pt.'s responses to medications & transfusions; monitor for side effects & toxic symptoms;
- encourage physical activity as tolerated & according to pt.'s ability; see NCPGs #2:26, "Aged Patient: Common Behaviors," & #2:32, "Aged Patient: Exercises;"
- if pt. is confined to bed, pay strict attention to skin condition, e.g., bathing, backrubs, change of position; (necessary to prevent skin breakdown); remember pt. is in a state of malnutrition & is a prime candidate for decubitis ulcers (refer to NCPG #4:42);
- administer mouth care after meals, snacks, & PRN.

3) Prevention of   The patient remains free of progression of disease; the patient is protected from sustaining accidents while in the
   Complic-   hospital:
   ations
- teach pt. to avoid very hot & very cold water or substances on hands, arms, legs, & feet in order to prevent trauma to skin due to decreased ability to perceive hot & cold;
- assess the effect of neurological impairment of pt.'s ability to do activities of daily living (ADL); monitor & help pt. PRN for safety, while encouraging as much independence as possible;
- observe for irritability or confusion; take precautions that pt. does not injure self or others;
- encourage & support the pt. to take vitamin B-12 injections, medications, & to eat his meals & snacks; continuously reinforce that B-12 & a highly nutritious diet will control his disease & prevent further symptomotology.

Discharge Planning and Teaching Objectives/Outcomes

1) (Patient/Family/Significant Other) Can describe cause of illness and treatment.
2) Has a realistic plan for receiving vitamin B-12 injections.
3) Outlines his dietary needs: foods high in iron, protein, and vitamins, and has a week's sample menu.
4) Understands neurological impairment limitations and has a plan to deal with these limitations at home.
5) Knows not to use hot water bottles or ice packs; states s/he will observe own extremities frequently and guard against hitting them against objects that s/he does not feel. Knows that own sensation for pain and heat are impaired.

Recommended References

"Anemias in the Elderly," by M.J. Clark-Williams. *Nursing Times*, March 3, 1977:299-301.

"Aged Patient: Common Behaviors." *NCP Guide* ©*2:26*, 2nd Ed., Nurseco, 1980.

"Aged Patient: Exercises for Patients Over 65." *NCP Guide* ©*2:32*, 2nd Ed., Nurseco, 1980.

"Decubitus Ulcer Care: Prevention and Treatment." *NCP Guide* ©*4:42*, Nurseco, 1978.

"Macrocytic Megaloblastic Anemias," by C. Wood. *Nurse Practitioner*, July/August 1977:33-35.

"The Patient Adapting to Chronic Illness Role." *NCP Guide* ©*5:30*, Nurseco, 1981.

"Test Yourself, Pernicious Anemia," by E. Robbins. *Nursing Mirror*, November 18, 1976:66-68.

The Patient with Radiation Implant/GYN

Definition: The insertion of radioactive materials into gynecological tissues for the purpose of destroying malignant cells.

LONG TERM GOAL: The patient will experience full therapeutic value from radiation implant treatment and will return to home/family/occupation with minimal physical and/or psychological untoward effects.

General Considerations:
- **Types of radioactive isotopes used:** Radium, iridium, phosphorus, gold, cesium, or iodine.
- **Types of internal radiation:** (1) *intracavitary* — applicators of isotopes placed inside body cavities, such as uterus; & (2) *interstitial* — isotope needles inserted into tissues, such as breast. Time is predetermined, but implantation may be temporary or permanent. It can also be placed in a mold or form for delivering dosage to small areas. Applicators may be "pre-loaded" in operating room before insertion or "after-loaded" in the patient's hospital room by a radiotherapist. The latter method exposes hospital personnel to less radiation.
- **Purpose** of radioactive implants is to retard or destroy malignant processes within accessible parts of the body. Implanted isotopes frequently are used in conjunction with other types of cancer therapy such as surgery, deep radiation, or chemotherapy.
- **Nursing responsibilities** include preoperative preparation and teaching of patient and postoperatively, (1) assessment of the patient's altered state of dependency and social isolation during restricted activity and visitors; (2) knowledge and precautionary activities regarding controls regulating family and personnel exposure to radiation; and (3) assessment, planning intervention, and evaluation of nursing measures to maintain bio/psycho/social well-being of patient with cancer. Refer to NCPG #2:07, "The Patient with Cancer: Early Stages."
- **Radiation exposure** can be minimized for caretakers by keeping in mind principles of *distance, shielding,* and *time.* The radiation received varies inversely (drops) with the square of the distance maintained from the source of radiation. Nurses should stay as far as possible from the patient when providing explanations or non-touch related nursing care. A lead shield should be used whenever possible. Keep the lead-insulated container or cart in the patient's room for immediately accessible use whenever radioactive material is removed or accidentally dislodged from the patient's body. Reduce the time spent with the patient by organizing work into short 15-20 minute segments, by planning ahead, and by working swiftly and efficiently. Wear film badge and pocket dosimeter near part of body most likely to receive greatest dosage. Turn in badge monthly and keep a

record of mrem exposure. US law requires persons who work near radiation sources to receive no more than 1250 millirems every 3 months to whole body. A legally required Radiation Safety Officer must investigate ways to reduce exposure when a person receives more than 400 mrem in a month. Pregnant or potentially pregnant personnel should not be assigned to these patients. Patients with sealed radiation sources should not be placed together in a room because this increases the exposure dose for nurses. Private rooms are desirable but a postmenopausal woman may, if necessary, be placed in the same room with a patient who has a radiation implant. Bed linens stained with the patient's body fluids are *not* radioactive when the patient is receiving implanted radiation through a sealed source. Refer to NCPG #5:48, "Radiation Therapy: General Principles."

Specific Considerations, Potential Patient Outcomes, and Nursing Actions:

1) Preoperative Preparation

The patient explains the nature and extent of her disease, the purpose of surgery, the use of radiation implants and expected effects, and the necessary care and precautions to be taken postoperatively; the patient expresses acceptance, confidence, and willingness to cooperate fully with this treatment:

- explain what will be done & what will be expected of pt.; explain precautions including isolation & limitation of visitors while radiation implants are in place; try to assuage fears after encouraging ventilation of them;
- give antiseptic douche as ordered;
- prevent incidental bladder irradiation by ensuring the pt.'s bladder is emptied prior to implantation or insert Foley catheter if ordered;
- prevent incidental bowel irradiation by administering cleansing enemas & low residue diet, as ordered;
- refer to NCPG #2:44, "General Preoperative Nursing Care."

2) Postoperative Measures

The patient maintains adequate cardiopulmonary, elimination, musculoskeletal and other normal body functions; the patient maintains adequate fluid and electrolyte balance, gastrointestinal function is restored, and the patient tolerates a clear, low-residue liquid to soft diet while radiation implant is in place; the patient is free of preventable complications:

- know that pt. will be on complete bed rest with head elevated only 10-15°; pt. will probably not be allowed to turn from side to side or onto abdomen; prop shoulders with pillows to relieve pressure; maintain pt. position conducive to most effective alignment of isotope implant & be sure pt. understands need to stay as placed;
- have pt. perform mild arm, leg, & foot exercises;
- take TPR & BP Q4H; report elevations above 38°C. (100.4°F);

— monitor parenteral fluids, if ordered; force fluids when oral intake allowed; record I&O accurately; notify physician of reduced intake, as dehydration is common;

— observe & report skin rash eruptions, vaginal discharge or excessive bleeding, abdominal distention or signs of dehydration;

— know & post clearly the precise time implant removal is ordered;

— see NCPGs #2:41, 42, 43, "General Postoperative Nursing Care, Parts A, B, & C," for additional appropriate nursing measures.

3) Relief of
   Pain

The patient will be as comfortable and pain-free as possible:

— observe pt. for non-verbal signs of pain & discomfort (restlessness, anxiety, irritability, increased pulse);

— inform pt. that intrauterine contractions should be expected with implants in the pelvic region & can be relieved with medication; pt. should be encouraged to notify staff & request analgesia or sedation; ask pt. to report type, location & intensity of pain;

— administer analgesia & sedation as liberally as ordered & needed.

4) Personal
   Hygiene

The patient achieves goals of personal hygiene and experiences satisfaction with personal care throughout restricted period of isotope implantation:

— observe for foul-smelling vaginal discharge & provide perineal cleansing & rinsing as needed; take care not to dislodge implant or move pt. excessively;

— use room deodorants PRN;

— feed or assist pt. to eat; cleanse face & hands & give oral hygiene before & after meals; know that this is important because pt. appetite is usually poor anyway;

— don't give pt. complete bed bath or complete back rub; wash upper half of body only except for necessary perineal care; avoid disturbing pt. with bed linen changes, using disposable bed pads to cover damp or soiled areas;

— use personal care time to socialize with pt., to counsel, teach or listen.

5) Isotope
   Radiation
   Precautions

The patient receives therapeutic radiation without endangering family, friends, or health care personnel:

— keep "Radiation In Use" caution sign conspicuously posted outside on pt.'s closed door;

— limit time spent by personnel with pt. to that which is reasonable & necessary; urge staff to carry out care as quickly as possible; help them plan ahead to save time;

— have personnel stand as far away as possible from the implant while giving care or talking with pt.; use a lead shield when possible;

— be sure that all care takers wear film badges or dosimeters, according to your hospital radiation dept. procedure;

— do not assign pregnant or possibly pregnant care givers to pt.;

— limit visitors to those over 18 & who are definitely not pregnant; have them sit at least 3, preferably 6, ft. from pt.'s bed & source of radiation; use a lead shield whenever possible; limit total visiting time over days of implant to a total of nine hours;

— inspect all linen, bed pads, & dressings to make certain radioactive source did not come out; dispose of them according to your hospital procedure (they are sometimes left in room until implant is removed);

— keep readily available lead-insulated container or cart in pt.'s room with long ring-necked sterile forceps and sterile gloves in the event of accidental dislodgement of isotope implant.

6) Removal of Sealed Radiation Source

The patient expresses understanding and demonstrates cooperation with the procedure to remove radium implant:

— notify gynecology resident, radiotherapist, or attending physician prior to the established time of removal, the exact removal time that has been ordered;

— pre-medicate pt. one hour before removal of radiation implant;

— have a sterile, long, ring forceps and sterile gloves ready at bedside;

— be certain that cart or lead transport carrier is available in room at bedside;

— explain procedure to pt. & answer any questions;

— drape pt. in lithotomy position;

— place pads & packing in plastic bag & arrange for correct disposal;

— collect sterile urine specimen & remove catheter, as ordered;

— after implant has been removed, record time of removal & catheter removal as well as pt. response; call radiation technician to pick up implant carrier;

— assist pt. to be up as desired, shower, & have visitors.

Discharge Planning and Teaching Objectives/Outcomes

1) Patient/Family/Significant Other) Is aware of amount and kind of care patient will need at home, and has verbalized confidence in a realistic arrangement or plan to provide it.

2) Has been referred to a home health agency, VNA, or other community nursing care resource; has phone number of local American Cancer Society.

3) Knows procedure for administering douches and how to prepare prescribed solution.

4) Knows that emollient enemas may relieve rectal irritation and knows how to administer these.

5) Knows to resume activities gradually over a period of weeks; to resume sexual intercourse when ready for it; and to balance rest with exercise.

6) Knows to avoid direct sunlight on skin areas exposed to radiation and that emollient cream or lotion can relieve dryness or itching.

7) Knows to observe and report promptly to physician any frequency, burning urination, diarrhea, nausea, vomiting, temperature over 100°F., and severe pain, as well as redness, warmth and tenderness in venipuncture sites or legs.

Recommended References

"Fatigue in Patients Receiving Localized Radiation," by Pamela Haylock and Laura Hart. *Cancer Nursing,* December 1979:461-467.

"General Postoperative Nursing Care, Part A, Part B, Part C." *NCP Guides #2:41, 42, 43,* 2nd Ed., Nurseco, 1980.

"General Preoperative Nursing Care." *NCP Guide #2:44,* 2nd Ed., Nurseco, 1980.

"Nursing Process and Chemotherapy for the Woman with Cancer of the Reproductive System," by Barbara Hildebrand. *The Nursing Clinics of North America,* June 1978:351-368.

"The Patient with Cancer: Early Stages." *NCP Guide #2:07,* 2nd Ed., Nurseco, 1980.

"Radiation Therapy: General Principles." *NCP Guide #5:48,* Nurseco, 1981.

"Radiation Therapy, Internal Radiation," by Kathleen Gillick. *Cancer Nursing,* August 1979:313-325.

"Working Safely Around Implanted Radiation Sources," by Mary Anne Breeding and Myron Wollin. *Nursing 76,* May 1976:59-63.

The Patient with a Salpingo/Ovariectomy (Oophorectomy)

Definition: Salpingo/ovariectomy (oophorectomy) is the excision and removal of an oviduct (tube) and ovary.

LONG TERM GOAL: The patient will return to her optimum level of health and resume usual roles in home, family, community after a normal, short convalescence; the patient will accept and cope effectively with her altered body image and loss.

General Considerations:

— **Indications:** to remove a ruptured ectopic pregnancy or other abnormal condition such as endomitriosis or a tumor; as an initial treatment of choice for pre-menopausal patients with metastatic breast cancer.

— **Consequences:** if both ovaries are removed, changes resulting from diminished estrogen secretion are noted (hot flushes, atrophied and pendulous breasts, less pubic hair). Psychological impact varies depending on the cause of surgery and its extent. Ambivalent feelings and emotional disturbances relating to loss may be observed. Fears include of dying, of cancer, of loss of femininity and sexuality, of pain, of loss of childbearing ability, of ability to cope or control destiny, and of weight gain or other menopausal changes. The reactions and attitudes of husband, family, and friends will affect the perceptions and the postoperative adjustment of the patient as well as the length of convalescence.

— **Preoperative nursing responsibility** is that for general abdominal surgery with the addition of a complete perineal prep and a cleansing douche as ordered; refer to NCPG #2:44, "General Preoperative Nursing Care." In addition, provide the patient with the information and reassurance she wants or needs re: hospitalization (less than a week), the operation, the expected postoperative course and convalescence. Nurses should be aware of what this operation means to patient so as to avoid inadvertent casualness or oversolicitude.

— **Postoperative nursing responsiblitiy** is similar to that for hysterectomy or abdominal surgery; refer to NCPGs #2:41, 42, 43, "General Postoperative Nursing Care, Part A, Part B, & Part C." In addition see NCPGs #1:12, "The Patient with a Hysterectomy" and #2:29, "The Patient Experiencing a Body Image Disturbance."

Specific Considerations, Potential Patient Outcomes, and Nursing Actions:

1) General Abdominal Surgery Postop Measures

The patient resumes normal cardiopulmonary function and fluid and electrolyte balance; the patient will be free of preventable complications; the patient will maintain adequate output and normal elimination will be restored:
- turn, cough, deep breathe pt. Q2H;
- monitor & record TPR & BP according to standard postop routine until stable;
- monitor & record parenteral fluids; record I&O carefully & accurately;
- administer antibiotics, vitamins & minerals, sedatives & analgesics as ordered; observe for untoward reactions — record & report;
- give food & fluids as tolerated when parenteral fluids are DCed & peristalsis returns;
- keep in low Fowler's or flat position to prevent increased & intra-abdominal pressure; apply abdominal binder for additional comfort & support;
- give passive & active leg exercises Q4H;
- if indwelling urethral catheter in place, see NCPG #2:39, "Catheters: Indwelling Urinary;" otherwise check voiding Q4H; measure amt. voided; notify Dr. if voiding frequent, small amts. or if unable to void in 6hrs. when intake has been adequate; observe for signs of bladder infection;
- check dressing for unusual bleeding; reinforce PRN; report accordingly; use strict aseptic technique when changing or handling dressings;
- note & report temperature elevations of two or more degrees after the third postoperative day;
- ambulate pt. according to orders, noting tolerance to activity.

2) Psychosocial Adjustment

The patient adapts effectively to trauma of surgery, to her loss and altered body image; the patient expresses growing confidence in ability to cope independently:
- provide regular opportunities for talking, asking questions, expressing feelings, & planning for the future;
- assess pt. feelings over loss (e.g., loss of pregnancy, or of ability to get pregnant in future); pt. may have ambivalent feelings (sad/glad); support ventilation of feelings & adaptive coping; see NCPG #1:31, "Responses to Loss: The Grief and Mourning Process;"
- assess pt.'s fears (e.g., of spread of cancer, of dying; of loss of sexuality & femininity); encourage pt. to ask questions; provide information PRN; refer to NCPG #1:28, "The Patient Experiencing Fear;"

— reinforce what doctor has told her about avoidance of heavy lifting, climbing stairs, driving, vacuuming (usually for at least ten days but may vary); about resumption of sexual intercourse; about return surgical appointment.

Discharge Planning and Teaching Objectives/Outcomes

1) (Patient/Family/Significant Other) Knows what surgery has been done and what changes in herself to expect (menopausal symptoms, weakness, fatigue, depression) during convalescence.
2) Knows to avoid sexual intercourse, heavy lifting, vacuuming, pushing a full grocery cart, driving or prolonged sitting for about ten days or as indicated by doctor.
3) Has written appointment, date, and time for follow-up visit to surgeon; understands care of incision; knows to call doctor for signs of illness, pain in abdomen, legs or chest, increased draining at incision site or a fever.

Recommended References

"Catheters: Indwelling, Urethral." *NCP Guide #2:39*, 2nd Ed., Nurseco, 1980.
"General Postoperative Nursing Care, Part A, Part B, Part C." *NCP Guides #2:41, 42, 43*, 2nd Ed., Nurseco, 1980.
"General Preoperative Nursing Care," *NCP Guide #2:44*, 2nd Ed., Nurseco, 1980.
"The Patient Experiencing a Body Image Disturbance." *NCP Guide #2:29*, 2nd Ed., Nurseco, 1980.
"The Patient Experiencing Fear." *NCP Guide #1:28*, 2nd Ed., Nurseco, 1980.
"The Patient with a Hysterectomy." *NCP Guide #1:12*, 2nd Ed., Nurseco, 1980.
"Responses to Loss: the Grief and Mourning Process." *NCP Guide #1:31*, 2nd Ed., Nurseco, 1980.

The Patient Undergoing Stapedectomy

Definition: Stapedectomy is the surgical removal of otosclerotic lesions of stapes and replacement with a prosthetic device to maintain conduction and ability to hear.

LONG TERM GOAL: The patient will recover free of complications and will express adequate knowledge of condition and treatment; the patient will return to usual roles in home/job/community while adhering to medical regimen.

General Considerations:

— Stapedectomy is done for otosclerosis, a condition in which there is a loss of hearing from gradual immobilization of the footplate of the stapes bone in the oval window of the ear. New growth of bone around the stapes blocks its movement so that it is no longer free to vibrate. Both ears are usually affected, not necessarily in equal degree.

— Otosclerosis is seen more frequently in women and becomes apparent in the 20s or 30s; first symptoms may include diminished hearing and a buzzing tinnitus (ringing in ears).

— After surgery, hearing usually improves, although it may not be experienced as "normal" hearing. Post-surgical complications may include sudden deafness from scar tissue formation or infection.

— **Nursing responsibilities** include:
  (1) preparing the patient for surgery, both physically and emotionally (see NCPG #2:44, "General Preoperative Care;")
  (2) ensuring that the patient has realistic expectations regarding outcomes; and
  (3) assessing patient's knowledge of surgical procedure and prognosis that hearing may not return immediately.

Specific Considerations, Potential Patient Outcomes, and Nursing Actions:

1) Prevention of Compli-cations

The patient will adapt to post-surgical regimen and recover free from complications;
— refer to NCPGs #2:41, 42, 43, "General Postoperative Care;"
— know & assist pt. to follow MD's orders for first 24 hours; these may include staying flat in bed, even for meals, keeping head movements to a minimum, moving slowly, avoiding blowing nose;
— position pt. as ordered; restricted head position may be ordered to maintain position of prosthesis & stability & promote draining;
— observe dressing for draining & reinforce PRN; instruct pt. to keep hands away from dressing;
— replace soiled cotton pledget in ear canal as surgeon orders, using aseptic technique;

— protect pt. from falling by using side rails, assist in ambulation; inform pt. that vertigo is a common occurrence & instruct to call for help with ambulation;

— observe & report signs of injury to facial nerve; ask pt. to pucker lips, close lips, wrinkle forehead; Inability to comply may mean nerve damage or edema causing pressure on nerve;

— observe & report symptoms of fever, headache, ear pain (may indicate infection, inner ear reaction);

— administer prescribed pain, sedative, or antiemetic medication as needed.

2) Psychosocial The patient will verbalize feelings and concerns related to surgical procedure to restore hearing.
   Adjustment   — approach in unhurried, calm manner to assess physical & emotional symptoms & needs;

— spend time listening to pt.'s concerns & feelings; pt. may be frustrated or depressed because hearing does not improve immediately; remind pt. that hearing may not improve for weeks.

— include family & significant other as pt. wishes; give *written* as well as verbal instructions for after-care & convalescent period;

— remember that both ears are usually affected & pt. may have hearing problem on ear which did *not* have surgical procedure.

Discharge Planning and Teaching Objectives/Outcomes

1) (Patient/Family/Significant Other) Has written appointment date and time for follow-up care with surgeon (ear packing usually removed 6th or 7th day in surgeon's office.)

2) Knows to reinforce or change outer ear dressing using aseptic technique; has demonstrated ability to do this.

3) Knows precautions of convalescence period such as: avoid sudden movements, elevators, flying in airplane and high altitudes; do not take showers, wash hair, swim, or get water on ear dressing; avoid crowds, people with respiratory infections, sudden head movements; close eyes when riding in traffic to prevent sudden head movements; do not smoke or blow nose (can cause irritation and scar tissue formation).

4) Knows to call surgeon immediately if pain or fever occur.

Recommended References
"General Preoperative Care." *NCP Guide #2:44*, 2nd Ed., Nurseco, 1980.
"General Postoperative Care." *NCP Guide #2:41, 2:42, 2:43*, 2nd Ed., Nurseco, 1980.

The Patient with a Tubal Ligation (via Mini-Laparotomy)

Definition: A tubal ligation via mini-laparotomy is a small incision between the navel and the pubis for the purpose of cutting the Fallopian tubes in half and tying them off.

LONG TERM GOAL: The patient will return to her optimum level of health and resume usual roles in home/family/community after a normal, short convalescence; the patient will accept and cope effectively with her altered body image and loss.

General Considerations:

— A form of permanent tubal sterilization; approximately 1-2 out of 1,000 could still get pregnant after this operation.

— **Indications:** multiparity, concomitant serious disease conditions, including inheritable conditions, socio-economic or other seriously considered reason for wanting to avoid pregnancy.

— **Legal Implications:** Most important factor is whether or not the woman has carefully considered the pros and cons of sterilization and has reached her informed decision independently without fear, pressure from others, or haste. Time should be provided by surgeon and nurse to answer all questions honestly and completely. A counselor should be consulted if patient indicates a need or desire to discuss issue with another professional person. If woman is married, the husband's permission must also be obtained. He should be given the same consideration as the wife to reach an informed decision alone. Written consents are obtained from both legally responsible persons. Compliance with the laws of state in which operation is performed is necessary.

— **Nursing responsibilities** are those for preoperative and postoperative care similar to patients having abdominal surgery, with some exceptions: A much smaller abdominal and perineal skin area is prepped, an enema and intravenous fluid are *not* given, and the patient may even be admitted and discharged on the day of surgery. A 12-24 hour hospitalization is common unless the patient has some complication. An antiseptic douche is given preoperatively and a brief explanation of the postoperative course is provided. Normally, the patient can return to her usual activities in a few days. Sometimes, however, a "bleeder" may occur during surgery that requires cauterization or a laparoscope may be used with carbon dioxide that may cause a "post-insufflation syndrome" of chest, neck, and shoulder pain. This may increase the convalescent period by a few days. Refer to NCPGs #2:44, "General Preoperative Nursing Care," #2:41, 42, 43, "General Postoperative Nursing Care, Part A, Part B, & Part C."

Specific Considerations, Potential Patient Outcomes, and Nursing Actions:

1) General Abdominal Surgery Postoperative Measures   The patient will resume normal cardio-pulmonary function with fluids and electrolytes in balance; the patient will be free of preventable complications; the patient will maintain adequate output with normal elimination restored:
   - turn, cough, deep breathe pt. Q2H;
   - monitor & record TPR & BP according to standard postop routine until stable;
   - monitor & record I&O carefully, accurately; give food & fluids as tolerated & as ordered;
   - administer analgesics PRN; assist pt. to sit up, dangle legs, & ambulate as soon as able & permitted;
   - check dressing for unusual bleeding; reinforce PRN, report accordingly; use strict aseptic technique when handling dressing & teach pt. this care.

2) Psychosocial Adjustment   The patient adapts effectively to this type of surgery and its resulting consequence of body image change:
   - since this surgery is usually elective, minor in its procedure & convalescence, & presumably desired by the pt., adaptation to the stress of hospitalization & surgery is expected and usually without discomfort psychologically; nevertheless, be careful of false assumptions re: pt.'s well-being; provide opportunities for talking, asking questions, expressing feelings, & resuming independence;
   - reinforce doctor's instructions about wound care, follow-up appt., return to work, & resumption of normal living activities (including sexual intercourse).

Discharge Planning and Teaching Objectives/Outcomes

1) (Patient/Family/Significant Other) Has written appointment (or number to call for one) for follow-up surgical office visit; can state information re: care of incision and activities permitted.
2) Knows to call doctor immediately for signs of illness: fever; pain in abdomen, legs or chest; increased draining at incision site or other untoward signs.

Recommended References

"General Postoperative Care. Parts A. B. and C." *NCP Guides #2:41, 42, 43*, 2nd Ed., Nurseco, 1980.
"General Preoperative Care." *NCP Guide #2:44*, 2nd Ed., Nurseco, 1980.

The Patient with Ulcerative Colitis

Definition: Ulcerative colitis is an inflammatory disease of the colon and rectum that results in ulceration, bleeding, and mucoid diarrhea.

LONG TERM GOAL: The patient will heal and regain normal bowel function; the patient will participate in medical regimen and lifestyle changes to prevent recurrence of symptoms.

General Considerations:
— **Incidence:** most common in young and middle-aged adults, slightly more in females,
— **Cause** is unknown although there is a familial tendency; usually several precipitating factors including stess, auto-immune factors, allergy, organisms causing infection, emotional responses that alter blood supply to colon mucosa causing ulceration.
— **Prognosis:** serious disease, often accompanied by systemic complications and a high mortality rate; 10% of patients develop carcinoma of colon. May be acute or in remission with chronic disease pattern.
— **Signs and symptoms:** cramping and severe diarrhea with blood and mucus in stool; fever, nausea and vomiting, anorexia, dehydration, weight loss, anemia, electrolyte imbalance; begins in rectum and spreads upward through colon,
— **Diagnostic evaluation:** stool exam, sigmoidoscopy, proctoscopy, barium enema x-ray (cathartic contraindicated).
— **Treatment** consists of three types: 1) care of acute exacerbations; 2) maintenance of remission; and 3) prevention of acute episodes and complications. Acute care includes medical regimen to reduce inflammation to suppress autoimmune responses, and to provide rest for diseased bowel so that it can heal. Psychotherapy is often utilized to assess for environmental factors that are stressors, to work with patient and family to modify stressors, and to learn new coping methods for stress. Surgery may be indicated to remove chronically-diseased segments of intestine and to maintain intestinal function through an ileostomy; refer to NCPG #1:13, "The Patient with an Ileostomy."
— **Nursing responsibilities** include 1) assessment, care, and evaluation of activities to promote effective healing of colon and to restore patient to optimal health; and 2) counseling with health teaching to enable the patient to accept and to participate in appropriate therapeutic regimen and modified lifestyle to prevent recurrence of ulcerative colitis.

Specific Considerations, Potential Patient Outcomes, and Nursing Actions:

1) Rest, Comfort and Relaxation

The patient experiences physical and mental rest in tension-reduced environment; the patient rests and allows intestinal tract to heal:
- reduce light, noise, unwelcome visitors & unnecessary stimuli in surroundings; plan care around regular rest periods;
- give sedatives & tranquilizers for rest & to allow peristalsis to slow down, thus resting bowel tract;
- turn Q2H when awake & position for comfort; be aware of possibility of skin breakdown; offer protective skin care pillows to relieve pressure & to provide support;
- give backrubs & teach muscle relaxation techniques to relieve tension; when out of acute phase, consider use of biofeedback, self-hypnosis, or transcendental meditation techniques to enable pt. to induce own state of relaxation; refer to NCPG #5:49, "Stress Management."

2) Control of Diarrhea

The patient's bowel movements are observed and recorded; the patient is free of cramping and diarrhea:
- observe & record bowel movements, noting frequency, time, amount, color, presence of blood or mucus, consistency (watery or semiformed); if possible, note presence of stress, visitors, or meal that may coincide with bowel movement;
- encourage pt. to participate in accurate intake & output recording; explain importance of recording bowel movements to assess patterns of progress or regression;
- report any evidence of sudden abdominal distention that could be symptom of megacolon or perforation;
- keep bedpan & wipes within reach if pt. is confined to bed; empty & clean bedpan immediately after each use;
- provide privacy & convenience in toilet facilities with an ample supply of soft toilet tissue, hygiene supplies of mild soap & water, & adequate linens; provide room deodorizer;
- give medications as ordered & observe for bowel movement changes.

3) Skin Integrity

The patient is free of skin breakdown and maintains skin integrity; the patient's skin and perianal area are clean, dry and odor free:
- provide meticulous perianal skin care to prevent & treat skin breakdown; keep perianal area clean, dry & odor free, using plain water on irritated or open areas, mild soap & water, powder or soothing lotion on surrounding areas;

    — observe skin over entire body & be aware of possibility of skin breakdown due to enforced inactivity & malnutrition; provide mouth care.

4) Nutrition, Fluids, and Electrolytes

The patient maintains adequate fluid and electrolyte balance; the patient ingests special diet to meet nutritional needs of body and to prevent irritation of inflamed colon:

— record intake & output carefully; monitor administration of parenteral fluids, electrolytes, & vitamin supplements; refer to NCPGs #2:46, "Intravenous Therapy, " & #3:48, 49, "Fluids and Electrolytes, Parts A & B;"

— know that these pts. are especially vulnerable to dehydration & electrolyte imbalance; watch for signs of potassium deficit (weakness, faint irregular pulse, paresthesias, soft flabby muscles) & sodium deficit (abdominal cramps, hypotension, rapid & thready pulse, apathy); refer to serum electrolyte reports & report promptly abnormal findings; see NCPG #2:48, "Potassium Imbalance;" consult with pt. & dietician to provide a well-balanced bland, low-residue, high-protein diet; assess which foods agree with pt. & which do not; modify diet plan accordingly; include foods high in electrolytes & low in fiber that pt. can tolerate; these may include bananas, potatoes (without skin), fish, strained fruit juice; see NCPG #5:40, "Diet: Low-Residue."

— advise pt. to avoid cold fluids that may increase gastric motility; mild, alcoholic beverages & spices should be avoided;

— encourage pt. to participate in planning for own nutrition needs to regain sense of power & some control over medical regimen & healing; see NCPG #5:34, "The Patient Experiencing Powerlessness;"

— avoid power struggle with pt. over diet; be matter of fact & let pt. learn choice & consequences of choices;

— if hyperalimentation therapy used, refer to NCPG #3:50, "Hyperalimentation."

5) Medications

The patient receives medications as ordered to manage symptoms and achieve remission of disease process; the patient is monitored for action and side effects of medications; the patient states action and symptoms of side effects to report to physician and nurse:

— administer medications as ordered; monitor & chart reaction; observe for side effects & report to physician; know that the medication regimen may include antichloinergics (to lessen cramps & diarrhea), sulfasalazine (for antibacterial & anti-inflammatory effects), broad spectrum antibiotics (to reduce secondary infections), adrenocorticosteroids (to inhibit the inflammatory reaction), vitamin & mineral supplements (to promote maximum healing);

— advise pt. taking sulfasalazine to drink at least 1,500ml of liquid daily to avoid kidney stone formation; inform patient that this drug may turn urine orange; observe & report side effects of anorexia, nausea, vomiting & gastric distress;

— know precautions & side effects of steroid drugs; give pt. antacid or food with drug to prevent gastric irritation; be aware that steroids can mask the symptoms of infection & thus promote its spread; report to Dr. immediately any pt. complaints of increasing illness or pain; note possible side effects of steroids: cushingoid features, obesity, hypertension, acne; see NCPG #5:43, "Drugs: Corticosteroids;" steroids may be given in the form of retention enemas to provide topical & symptomatic relief;

— inform pt. of action of medications as well as symptoms & side effects to report to nurse & physician;

— expect drug dosage to be decreased by physician as symptoms improve & remission is achieved.

6) Psychosocial Adjustment

The patient experiences a trust relationship with nursing staff; the patient expresses feelings, fears and concerns to a receptive professional person; the patient participates in assessing for stressors and planning lifestyle change to cope with stress and prevent activation of disease process:

— spend time at beginning of shift to assess pt.'s needs & concerns, & to plan interventions around rest periods; build trust relationship by listening, offering respect & support, meeting pt.'s immediate needs; offer hope & encouragement;

— assess level of anxiety & discomfort; know that chronic diarrhea causes emotional & physical debilitation, with depression, discouragement, & powerlessness;

— encourage pt. to express feelings, fears, & concerns; accept anger & frustration & support pt. in taking sick role in acute phase; see NCPG #5:36, "The Patient Adapting to the Sick Role;"

— offer caring & support of dependency needs; recognize that psychotherapy in acute phase may do more harm than good; see NCPG #1:25, "The Patient Manifesting Dependency;"

— encourage pt. to participate in planning & evaluating own care; give choices whenever possible in activities of daily living, rest periods, meal schedules, visiting hours;

— set limits as necessary; contract with pt. within time frame for realistic care plan; be dependable (example: plan for AM care 7:30, breakfast 8:00, rest period 8:30-9:30, bath at 9:30, rest period 10:30-11:30, with pt. to use call light only if necessary); see NCPG #1:29, "The Patient Manifesting Manipulation;"

— when acute phase is over & pt. experiences remission of symptoms, assess pt.'s knowledge of ulcerative colitis as a chronic illness pattern & health teach precipitating factors of acute episodes, diet adaptations, medication administration, rest & exercise, importance of prevention; see NCP Guide #5:30, "The Patient Adapting to Chronic Illness Role;"

— assess for stressors in environment & lifestyle; problem solve with pt. to explore potential lifestyle changes to cope with stress more effectively & to prevent activation of disease process; utilize role playing, assertion training, communication techniques, relaxation.

Discharge Planning and Teaching Objectives/Outcomes

1) (Patient/Family/Significant Other) Can state basic facts of ulcerative colitis: signs and symptoms of acute phase, precipitating factors, medical treatment.
2) Has written outline of physician's recommendations for diet, rest and exercise, stress reduction, and relaxation.
3) Has received written instructions for medications to take home and can state dosage, frequency, action, and possible side effects to report to physician.
4) Can state importance of follow-up visit to physician to evaluate healing process, monitor medical regimen and psychosocial adjustment.

Recommended References

"Are You Prepared for Your Ulcerative Colitis Patient?" by Kristine Koner. *Nursing 80*, April 1980:43-35.
"Diet: Low-Residue." NCP Guide #*5:41*, Nurseco, 1981.
"Durgs: Corticosteroids." *NCP Guide #5:43*, Nurseco, 1981.
"Fluids & Electrolytes, Parts A & B." *NCP Guide #3:48, 49*, Nurseco, 1977.
"Hyperalimentation." *NCP Guide #3:50*, Nurseco, 1977.
"Intravenous Therapy." *NCP Guide #2:46*, 2nd Ed., Nurseco, 1980.
"The Patient Adapting to Chronic Illness Role." *NCP Guide #5:30*, Nurseco, 1977.
"The Patient Adapting to the Sick Role." *NCP Guide #5:36*, Nurseco, 1981.
"The Patient Experiencing Powerlessness." *NCP Guide #5:43*, Nurseco, 1981.
"The Patient with an Ileostomy." *NCP Guide #1:13*, 2nd Ed., Nurseco 1980.
"The Patient Manifesting Dependency." *NCP Guide #1:25*, 2nd Ed., Nurseco, 1980.
"The Patient Manifesting Manipulation." *NCP Guide #1.29*, 2nd Ed., Nurseco, 1980.
"Potassium Imbalance." *NCP Guide #2:48*, 2nd Ed., Nurseco, 1980.
"Stress Management." *NCP Guide #5:49*, Nurseco, 1981.

The Patient with a Vulvectomy

Definition: Vulvectomy is the surgical excision of the external female genitalia consisting of the labia majora, labia minora, and clitoris.

LONG TERM GOAL: The patient will recover from surgery, accept an altered body image, and return to usual roles in home, job, community after a normal convalescence with a minimum of physical/psychological complications.

General Considerations:
- **Indications:** chronic leukoplakia and/or cancer of the vulva.
- **Incidence:** 2-3% of all women over fifty, peaking in women of the mid-sixties age.
- **Signs and symptoms:** white, thickened skin in vulvar area that itches and is susceptible to chronic inflammation, irritations, sores, fissures. Unusual discharge, bleeding, skin rash, or lumps may be present.
- **Treatment:** After complete physical and history, biopsy and determination of presence of metastases, a simple or hemivulvectomy may be indicated. If more extensive surgery is required, a radical vulvectomy is done along with bilateral, inguinal node dissection and, if needed, resection of the vagina, urethra, and bowel. Radiation therapy and plastic reconstruction surgery may be performed after the initial vulvectomy recovery period.
- **Nursing responsibilities** include those for "General Preoperative Nursing Care," (NCPG #2:44) and "General Postoperative Nursing Care," (NCPG s #2:41, 42, 43). In addition, the nurse plays an active role in assisting the patient and family to accept an altered body image and to adjust to the psychological impact of cancer and its treatment. Problems also may arise that are related to concomitant medical conditions frequently seen in women of this age; refer to the appropriate topics in the Nursing Care Planning Guide series.

Specific Considerations, Potential Patient Outcomes, and Nursing Actions:

1) Preoperative Preparation   The patient understands nature and extent of disease and surgery; the patient is actively engaged in adaptive process toward accepting an altered body image; the patient is informed about the general postoperative course, equipment, and treatment; the patient is physiologically and psychologically stabilized and prepared for surgery:
- provide explanations as needed & desired, being careful not to overwhelm pt. at any one time; repeat information as necessary; encourage pt. to express feelings about disfiguring, defeminizing type of surgery &

concerns about cancer, dying, pain; pt. may commonly try to hide feelings, avoid complaining & be a "good" pt.; help pt. to ventilate fear, anger, anxiety;
— provide complete skin prep, antiseptic douches, cleansing enemas & low-residue diet (to reduce perineal straining postoperatively) as prescribed;
— see NCPG #2:44, "General Preoperative Nursing Care," for additional actions;
— see NCPG #2:07, "The Patient with Cancer: Early Stages," for psychosocial interventions.

2) Postoperative Measures

The patient maintains adequate cardiopulmonary, elimination, musculoskeletal and other normal body functions; the patient maintains adequate fluid and electrolyte balance, regains normal gastrointestinal function, tolerates and progresses from a clear liquid to a normal diet; the patient is free of preventable complications of hemorrhage, infection, and venous thrombosis:
— irrigate the vulval wound periodically with prescribed antiseptic solution; keep the wound clean, dry, & free of rectal contamination; use sterile technique;
— position pt. to prevent tension on taut suture lines & further trauma to remaining friable vulva tissue;
— turn, cough, deep breathe pt. Q2H; demonstrate & monitor IPPB treatments; teach pt. to use "blow" bottles effectively;
— remove anti-embolic stockings or elastic bandages Q8H, then replace; provide passive, then active, leg exercises;
— provide adequate pain relief to prevent unnecessary restlessness & anxiety;
— be aware of dysuria potential after removal of catheter (edema & perineal tightening make voiding a problem); see NCPG #2:39, "Catheters: Indwelling, Urethral;"
— check vital signs according to standard post-op procedure; observe & record signs of hemorrhage, infection, or other untoward developments; note those symptoms appropriate to concomitant medical conditions of *this* pt.; empty & record bloody drainage from Hemovac or other suction device;
— monitor IV fluids & keep accurate I&O records until pt. progresses to a clear liquid, then regular, diet; see NCPG #2:46, "Intravenous Therapy;"
— see NCPGs #2:41, 42, 43, "General Postoperative Nursing Care," for additional nursing measures.

3) Psychosocial Adjustment

The patient demonstrates an active, adaptive process to accept altered body image, actively participates in a rehabilitative program, expresses negative feelings and constructively channels the associated energy by increasing self-care and decision-making activities:

- observe for signs of anger, revulsion, growing quietude, depression; spend time with pt. that is not spent entirely on physical care; encourage pt. to cry if she has been holding back; provide opportunity for pt. to establish trust & rapport with at least one nurse in order to encourage ventilation of feelings;
- arrange for diversional activities & people that provide pleasure for pt.; encourage socialization with other pts. & phone calls or visits from family & friends; explain & discuss the pt.'s adjustment with close, caring persons; ask them to support the pt.'s efforts to cope & adapt;
- teach pt. wound care & home convalescence measures (rest, exercise, diet, medications, resumption of sexual relations varies, 2-3mos.);
- begin to prepare pt. for further surgery, if reconstructive repair is scheduled, or for adjunct therapy of radiation treatments, if planned;
- see NCPG #2:07, "The Patient with Cancer: Early Stages" for additional measures; refer also to NCPG #2:29, "The Patient Experiencing a Body Image Disturbance."

4) Adjunct Therapy

The patient understands and adjusts to additional therapies indicated by the disease process; the patient is helped to cope with side effects of treatments; the patient expresses optimism and hope that life will be prolonged and improved as a result of treatments:

- provide information & reassurance to pt. on adjunct therapy selected; allow time for absorption of information, expressions of feelings & attitudes;
- provide privacy & assistance needed both physically & psychologically to attain optimum benefits of therapy;
- observe & record all pt. reactions to treatment as well as methods used to alleviate discomforts;
- protect pt. from exposure to infection by visitors, staff or other pts. with protective isolation procedures standard for your hospital;
- for additional nursing measures appropriate in radiation therapy and/or chemotherapy, refer to NCPG #2:07, "The Patient with Cancer: Early Stages," & NCPG #5:14, "The Patient with Pelvic Radiation."

Discharge Planning and Teaching Objectives/Outcomes

1) (Patient/Family/Significant Other) Demonstrates positive adaptation to altered body image through active participation in rehabilitation and self-care program with growing confidence.

2) Knows to recognize and report possible complications (signs of illness, increased bleeding) promptly; has appointment for follow-up medical supervision.

3) Has information about, and access to, community resources for physical, emotional and/or financial assistance during rehabilitation period.

4) Demonstrates acceptance of malignant process, arrested or incurable; returns to home/job/community with positive attitude and efforts toward independence.

Recommended References

"Catheters: Indwelling, Urethral." *NCP Guide #2:39*, 2nd Ed., Nurseco, 1980.

"Easing the Shock of a Radical Vulvectomy," by Diane Servatius. *Nursing 75*, August 1975:27-31.

"Fatigue in Patients Receiving Localized Radiation," by Pamela Haylock and Laura Hart. *Cancer Nursing*, December 1979:461-467.

"General Postoperative Nursing Care, Part A, Part B, Part C." *NCP Guides #2:41, 42, 43*, 2nd Ed., Nurseco, 1980.

"General Preoperative Nursing Care." *NCP Guide #2:44*, 2nd Ed., Nurseco, 1980.

"Intravenous Therapy." *NCP Guide #2:46*, 2nd Ed., Nurseco, 1980.

"Nursing Process and Chemotherapy for the Woman with Cancer of the Reproductive System," by Barbara Hildebrand. *The Nursing Clinics of North America*, June 1978:351-368.

"The Patient Experiencing a Body Image Disturbance." *NCP Guide #2:29*, 2nd Ed., Nurseco, 1980.

"The Patient with Cancer: Early Stages." *NCP Guide #2:07*, 2nd Ed., Nurseco, 1980.

"The Patient with Pelvic Radiation." *NCP Guide #5:14*, Nurseco, 1981.

The Child with Cerebral Palsy

Definition: Cerebral palsy is permanent, nonprogressive damage to a portion of the brain that results in neuromuscular disabilities or difficulty controlling voluntary muscles.

LONG TERM GOAL: The patient and family will accept and adjust to disabilities; the patient will develop and maintain abilities to function independently in self-care activities and will cooperate with plan to prevent complications and deformities.

General Considerations:
- **Incidence:** an estimated 25,000 babies are born with cerebral palsy in the United States annually (1.5 to 5 per 1000 live births).
- **Causes** include:
  - *problems with development in utero*: Rh factor, rubella in first trimester, ABO incompatability;
  - *complications at birth*: anoxia to brain due to trauma, prematurity with precipitate delivery; and
  - *problems of early childhood*: meningitis, encephalitis, poisoning, trauma to brain.
- Child may have normal or superior intelligence; if there is damage to cognitive area of brain, symptoms of mental retardation will be present.
- Multiple handicaps are common and may include speech or hearing impairment, mental retardation, convulsive disorders, and oculomotor impairment.
- **Types and descriptions:**
  - *Spastic* (50-70%): increased muscle tone with exaggerated, deep tendon reflexes; spasticity may involve all extremities, the legs only, or one side of the body. May have talipes equinus (walk on toes). Speech and swallowing may be impaired and child may drool constantly; child is more likely to be mentally retarded.
  - *Dyskinesia* (20-25%): athetoid movements (slow, writhing, wormlike) of extremities, head, and neck, increase under pressure or stress and decrease during sleep. Drooling may be excessive. Incidence of accompanying hearing loss is high.
  - *Ataxia* (1-10%): incoordination due to disturbance in sense of balance, posture, kinesthetic feedback, produces an unsteady, wide-based gait.
  - *Mixed* (15-40%): Usually some combination of spasticity with dyskinesia; *sometimes* ataxia with dyskinesia.
- **Early symptoms:** *in newborn*, include absence of normal reflexes, irritability, feeding problems, poor motor development, poor muscle tone; infant at risk is "small for date," premature, has complication with birth. (Check for infant spasticity by pushing

the baby's head forward; the baby with cerebral palsy will resist and push against your hand. Flex baby's legs onto abdomen and quickly release them; spastic legs will spring back into extension and then adduction with crossing or scissoring.)
- **Treatment**: usually a team effort for early diagnosis of specific disability with immediate initiation of infant-stimulation measures and therapeutic interventions to develop child's abilities and to prevent complications and deformities. The multidisciplinary team may include pediatrician, neurologist, physical therapist, speech therapist, nurse, social worker, and family members. The child and family are important team members and should be included and considered in planning, implementing, and evaluating treatment plan. The child with cerebral palsy may be admitted to acute hospital for orthopedic surgery to release contractures so that bracing and walking is possible, or for acute care of medical/surgical conditions.
- **Nursing responsibilities** include early detection of symptoms and reporting them to physician; working within an interdisciplinary team to assess, plan, implement, and evaluate individual treatment plan; and health teaching and counseling with patient and family.

Specific Considerations, Potential Patient Outcomes, and Nursing Actions:

1) Psychosocial Adjustment — The patient and family express in their own words an understanding of the disability; the patient/family cooperates with a plan for independent functioning and prevention of complications and deformities; the patient/family express feelings and concerns about limitations of function due to disability:
   - approach pt./family in calm, respectful, & unhurried manner; attitudes of acceptance, friendliness, & willingness to listen will promote a trust relationship;
   - assess pt./family members' level of understanding & acceptance of disability; be available to listen to feelings & concerns & accept expressed feelings in nonjudgmental way; refer to NCPG #3:29, "The Parent Experiencing Grief & Loss;"
   - offer emotional support as pt./family go through periods of adjustment & grief & mourning; a family member with cerebral palsy implies numerous problems & adjustments in daily life of the whole family, with constant demands, few rewards, & many frustrations;
   - offer hope that pt. can learn to be independent in activities of daily living (ADL) & can grow & develop abilities to adapt to limitations; know & inform family that although damage cannot be cured, new patterns can be established to enhance the quality of life of pt. & family;

- allow parent to be the expert on care of pt.; give acknowledgment & positive reinforcement to efforts to provide a stimulating, healthy environment & for parents' observation & abilities to assess pt.'s needs & provide for them; know that while practical advice & suggestion is important, the parent may feel inadequate & overwhelmed;
- ask parent to define concerns & problems; find out how long s/he has tried specific approach, how the approach works & does not work, what alternatives s/he already knows *before* giving suggestions or teaching; refer to NCPGs #3:32, "Teaching the Parent/Guardian/Child: General Suggestions," & #5:47, Problem Solving;"
- if the pt. has mental retardation, refer to NCPGs #4:21 & 22, "The Child with Developmental Disability: Mental Retardation."

2) Activities of Daily Living (ADL)

The patient performs ADL as independently as possible with the use of support measures as needed; the patient ingests adequate food and fluid to meet body needs:

- assess pt.'s preadmission level of functioning; obtain information from pt./family/care giver; know that an accurate assessment of pain & bodily needs is critical to ensure adequate food & fluid, as well as minimal pain;
- adjust hospital routine to pt.'s usual routine as much as possible; provide sameness & consistency in nursing care as pt. will respond better to exact schedules & time frames;
- allow time for pt. to participate in planning own care; assess strengths & help only as needed; utilize support measures (braces, special hygiene & eating utensils) that allow pt. to function independently in self-care activities; refer to NCPG #5:34, "The Patient Experiencing Powerlessness," for measures to increase independence & decrease powerlessness;
- allow time for pt. to be as independent as possible with ADL, especially with hygiene routines, mealtimes, ambulation;
- ensure adequate intake of food & fluid; if pt. uses special feeding utensils, make sure that they are present at mealtime; allow choice in menu when possible & use supplements as needed; provide privacy as needed if excessive drooling is a problem at mealtime;
- preserve skin integrity by massage, bathing, use of lotions, sheepskins, water mattress, etc.; bathe in warm water (cold or hot will trigger spasms);

    — use passive & active range of motion exercises as tolerated (see NCPG #1:47); provide rest periods & reduce stimuli to promote calm environment;

    — explain & demonstrate use of support systems such as suctioning, IVs, etc., in advance to decrease anxiety & increase cooperation;

    — give praise, verbal & nonverbal positive reinforcement for pt.'s abilities to function independently in self-care activities; see NCPG #5:37, "Behavior Modification."

3) Prevention of Complications and Deformities

The patient is free of preventable complications and deformities; the patient and family describe and demonstrate measures to promote maintenance of independent function and prevent complications and deformities:

    — protect from accidents resulting from poor balance & lack of muscle control; be aware that pt. may not be able to ask for help & may need to rely on nurse's assessment & judgment on what safety precautions are appropriate; do not wait for call light; plan regular, frequent checks of pt. condition, saftey rails up, etc.;

    — use seatbelts in wheelchairs & secure pt. in chair & bed as needed for safety;

    — observe for restlessness, agitation, dyspnea (may be indicative of fever or infection); know that pt. is susceptible to respiratory tract infections due to poor control of intercostal muscles & diaphragm; observe for choking or aspiration; remain with pt. until medications are safely swallowed;

    — measure & record I&O, note BM consistency & frequency, urine specific gravity, to ensure dehydration is not occurring; follow usual bowel & bladder training schedule so that pt. does not regress while in hospital;

    — note problems with hearing loss or blindness, speech or communication problems, or seizure precautions on care plan; notify others with sign at pt. bedside, according to hospital procedure;

    — work with physical therapist & family to ensure that active & passive ROM & usual exercise routine is followed as permitted by physical condition (to prevent contractures);

    — refer to NCPGs for medical & surgical conditions that apply to pt.

Discharge Planning and Teaching Objectives/Outcomes

1) (Patient/Family/Significant Other) Can demonstrate technical skills/procedures to be carried out after discharge and has adequate amount of supplies (dressing, etc.) to do so.

2) Has a written list of medications, dosage, and times to be taken; can describe actions & side effects that should be reported to physician.

3) Has an appointment for follow-up with physician/clinic, and a referral to a community support agency as appropriate.

4) Can describe and utilize services for patients and families provided by local branch of United Cerebral Palsy Association (national headquarters: 66 East 34 Street, New York, NY 10016).

5) Can describe in own words the rights of the handicapped, including educational opportunities with peers, availability to transportation and access to public places.

Recommended References

"Behavior Modification." *NCP Guide #5:37*, Nurseco, 1981.

"The Child with a Developmental Disability: Mental Retardation (in an Acute Setting)." *NCP Guide #4:22*, Nurseco, 1978.

"The Child with a Developmental Disability: Mental Retardation (in a Residential Setting)." *NCP Guide #4:22*, Nurseco, 1978.

"The Parent Experiencing Grief & Loss." *NCP Guide #3:29*, Nurseco, 1977.

"The Patient Experiencing Powerlessness." *NCP Guide #5:34*, Nurseco, 1981.

"Problem Solving." *NCP Guide #5:47*, Nurseco, 1981.

"Range of Motion Exercises." *NCP Guide #1:47*, 2nd Ed., Nurseco, 1980.

"Symposium of Central Nervous System Disorders in Children: Cerebral Palsy," by G.T. Davis et al. *Nursing Clinics of North America*, March 1980:35-50.

"Teaching the Parent/Guardian/Child: General Suggestions." *NCP Guide #3:32*, Nurseco, 1977.

The Child with Cleft Lip and Cleft Palate

Definition: Cleft lip and cleft palate are bilateral or unilateral congenital defects in the neonate.

LONG TERM GOAL: The parents will resolve feelings of producing a less-than-perfect newborn; the parents will learn to love and adequately care for the baby/child as s/he grows and develops; the parents will adapt to the need for years of treatment of the child's defect. The infant/child will receive adequate nutrition for growth and development; the infant/child will receive optimal treatment for congenital defect.

General Considerations:
- Cleft lip occurs when there is failure of the fissure of the lip to close; cleft palate results from incomplete closure of the maxillary process, the hard and soft palate may be involved or the soft palate alone. Cleft palate usually occurs with cleft lip; the cleft lip may occur alone.
- **Causes:** genetic or environmental factors while in utero such as drugs or viral infections. Both sexes affected equally. A cleft in the left lip is more prevalent than in the palate.
- Development of motor, psychological, and activity levels are usually normal in the clefted child.
- Middle ear effusion is present in the newborn infant with cleft palate, and is usually gone by age 5; there is a high incidence of middle ear infection and hearing loss.
- Clefted individuals drop from secondary school at a higher rate than non-clefted individuals. More clefted people remain single than in the general population. Though these individuals have the same needs as others, it is clear that their defects interfere in attaining goals and in developing satisfying relationships with others.
- **Treatment for cleft lip:** Surgical lip repair is usually performed during the first few weeks of birth when the baby is well hydrated, nourished, and in satisfactory health.
- **Treatment for cleft palate:**
  - X-rays are taken before surgery to help the surgeon plan his corrective measures.
  - Hard palate surgical repair can be done at 10 months of age; soft palate repair is done when maxillary structures are more fully developed, usually at 18-24 months of age.
  - Bone grafts for the hard palate may be taken from rib, tibia, or iliac crest; secondary grafts in adolescence may be required with usually good results.
  - More surgery may be required in adolescence when oral and facial structures increase dramatically in size.

- Sometimes a hard palate prosthesis is prescribed in place of surgery or until surgery can be done.
- Speech therapy is helpful to improve articulation and improvement of the acoustic product.
- Orthodontia in childhood is required to correct malocclusion.
- Long-term follow-up is required; the ideal team includes otolaryngologist, audiologist, pediatrician, nurse, social worker, radiologist, and speech therapist/pathologist.
- **Nursing responsibilities** at birth include helping the parents accept and adjust to their newborn with congenital defect(s) and teaching them to feed and care for their baby; preoperative preparation includes assessment of infant's physical status, preparation of the infant for surgery, and assistance for parents to cope psychologically with the stress of surgery to their child. Postoperative nursing responsibilities include: assessing the infant's responses after surgery and anesthesia, helping parents and child cope with the pain and discomfort, and instructing parents in proper care of their child. Refer to NCPGs #3:22, "Normal Growth & Development: Newborn" and #3:23, "Normal Growth & Development: Infant."

Specific Considerations, Potential Patient Outcomes, and Nursing Actions:

1) Care of the Newborn with Cleft Defect

The parents accept the infant with defects and are able to feed and care for him:

- allow the parents to express their negative feelings towards the baby; be aware that they were expecting a healthy baby & not a baby with a visible defect; give them acceptance & support;
- refer to NCPG #1:31, "Responses to Loss;" remember that the parents are grieving the loss of their expected perfect child;
- spend time with the parents, & be an attentive listener; introduce the fact that with surgery & a period of time the child's defect will be corrected; teach the parents that their newborn has the same needs as others to be fed, to be held, to be kept warm & dry; teach both parents to change & hold their newborn; point out positive aspects, e.g., color of hair, eyes, long fingers, tiny feet;
- ensure adequate nutrition for baby; prop the baby's head higher than his body with a pillow; feed the baby with a spoon, cup, or nipple specially designed for clefted babies; explain to the mother & father that the baby has trouble sucking because of the cleft; demonstrate feeding techniques to them & supervise them feeding baby;
- burp or bubble the baby frequently since s/he swallows large amount of air while feeding;
- if a maxillary prosthesis is used (it covers the cleft in palate), it should be removed and cleaned daily;
- praise the parents for their efforts at feeding; encourage the holding & feeding of the baby in a relaxed manner

since s/he is very responsive to parental anxiety;
- teach the parents that upper respiratory infections are common in clefted babies, & to notify their doctor of any fever over 101°, excessive mucous, diarrhea, or other symptoms distressing to the baby.

2) Postoperative Care

The baby is free of preventable complications from surgery; has adequate nutrition; the family demonstrates correct care of the baby:
- observe for bleeding & excess mucous in the mouth; maintain patent airway;
- keep suture line clean & dry; if suction is ordered, keep catheter away from suture line;
- use elbow splints to prevent baby from touching his sutures; remove splints one at a time QH to exercise arms; sometimes a special bar may be taped to the baby's face to go over the lip & prevent the baby from rubbing his lip on the sheets; babies squirm around a great deal, so be sure to observe & position so that s/he does not injure suture line;
- prevent pt. contact with persons with upper respiratory diseases;
- turn frequently (at least Q2H) from side to side, but *not on abdomen* (to protect suture line);
- feed baby with an asepto syringe with a rubber tip to prevent sucking & avoid tension on the suture line;
- tell mother that when suture line is healed, baby may return to previous method of feeding;
- encourage & assist parents to participate in the care of their infant when in the hospital: feeding, bathing, holding.

3) Preoperative Preparation for Repair of Cleft Palate

Infant is infection-free; the child is able to hold and drink from a cup:
- advise mother that she must teach child to drink from a cup in preparation for feeding after surgery; provide assistance PRN;
- inform mother to report a cold or other upper respiratory infection to the doctor immediately in the week prior to surgery (may be postponed for child's safety).

4) Postoperative Care of Repair Cleft Palate

The baby is free of preventable complications; the baby is adequately nourished; the family demonstrates correct care of the baby:
- observe for bleeding & excess mucous; report to Dr. PRN;
- keep airways clean; avoid touching sutures in palate during suction or feeding; turn from side to side Q2H;
- use restraints PRN so that child will not stick fingers or other objects in mouth; remove restraints one at a time every hour to exercise arms;

- prevent pt. contact with persons with upper respiratory infections;
- feed child a liquid diet *with a cup* until the suture line is healed; prevent sucking or use of a straw; as palate heals, child can be fed a soft, then regular, diet;
- allow mother to room in with child & to provide care: feeding, holding, bathing; know that this is particularly important at this age since separation anxiety from the mother is a consideration (refer to NCPG #3:20, "The Child with Separation Anxiety").

Discharge Planning and Teaching Objectives/Outcomes

1) (Family/Significant Other) Demonstrates correctly how to feed and care for the infant; knows infant's needs for love and security.
2) Has phone number to call if needs assistance with feeding, e.g., pediatrician or public health nurse.
3) Has a list of medications and special instructions for care of the infant; knows signs of infection (fever, runny nose, lethargy) and to report these to the doctor promptly.
4) Knows what plans have been made for correction of defect, specifically for the next 6 months and generally after that.
5) Has a referral to federal and local agencies that offer financial support for children with congenital defects.

Recommended References

"Bonding Problems of Infants with Congenital Anomalies," by E. Waechter. *Nursing Forum*, 16 3-4, 1977:298-318.
"The Care and Management of the Newborn Cleft Palate Infant," by A. Huddart. *Nursing Mirror*, January 1975:61.
"The Child with Separation Anxiety." *NCP Guide #3:20*, Nurseco, 1977.
"Crisis: a Baby Born with a Defect," by R. Mercer. *Nursing 77*, November 1977:45-47.
"Normal Growth & Development: Newborn." *NCP Guide #3:22*, Nurseco, 1977.
"Normal Growth & Development: Infant." *NCP Guide #3:23*, Nurseco, 1977.
"Nursing Care of the Infant and Child with Cleft Lip and Palate," by C. Sanchez. *Viewpoint*, January 1980:14-15.
"Responses to Loss: The Grief and Mourning Process." *NCP Guide #1:31*, 2nd Ed., Nurseco, 1980.
"Three into One will Go," by A. Mayman. *Nursing Mirror*, January 1979:31-33.

The Child's Conception of Death

LONG TERM GOAL: The child will express ideas and feelings about death; the child will learn to cope adaptively with loss and death.

General Considerations:
- The **development of a concept of death** takes place in stages that are interconnected with the normal sequence of biological and psychological growth. Children's concepts about death are more closely related to mental development and maturity than to chronological age; each child is unique with own special growth process and needs.
- A **child's behavior in response to death,** anticipated threat of loss of a loved one, and knowledge of own mortality is determined by a combination of variables including *concept development* according to maturity and cognitive ability, *socialization* into specific cultural and religious patterns of bereavement, and *life experiences* with death, dying, and life-threatening situations.
- **Children learn to cope** with death by observing attitudes and actions of parents, family, and friends; emotional support and health teaching with parents promotes adaptive coping with death in both child and parent. Children who are exposed to death and loss in a matter-of-fact, nonfrightening way tend to be less fearful and cope more adaptively with death and loss, compared to those who have not had this exposure.
- **Nursing responsibilities** include: (1) assessment of behaviors to determine concepts about death, influencing variables, and ability to cope; (2) planning and implementing interventions of health teaching and emotional support for child and parent; (3) self-assessment of own concepts and feelings about death and loss, knowledge of conceptual stages, behaviors, and nursing implications; and (4) utilization of a professional support system to integrate theory into practice and increase own ability to cope adaptively with death and loss in order to increase effectiveness and avoid stress and overload.

Childs Conception of Death According to Age.	Nursing Implications
1) **Infant and toddler:** believed to have no concept of death; are sensitive to parents' reactions, i.e., anxiety, anger, sadness, crying. If parent is upset, infant becomes upset.	— Assist parents to deal with their feelings about loss & death; this will allow them to build up emotional reserve to meet the needs of the infant. Refer to NCPGs #1:31, "Responses to Loss: The Grief and Mourning Process," & #3:29, "The Parent Experiencing Grief & Loss."

At age six to eight months, infant cries when recognizes strange, unknown face; this is called "stranger anxiety" and continues until end of first year.

Toddler cannot comprehend absence of life; may repeat "Grandpa's dead & gone to heaven" and still expect Grandpa to come to dinner. Ritual daily schedule important; may want to set dinner place for Grandpa or save chair for him.

Separation anxiety when parents leave or when toddler anticipates parents leaving continues from six months to six years.
Toddler is curious and concerned about sad feelings in parents, friends, and family members.

2) **Three to five year old:** may be more curious than concerned; views death as reversible and assumes dead can return. Primary fear is separation from mother or primary care taker. May associate death with sleep or absence of movement.

— Discuss "stranger anxiety" as normal developmental behavior *before* behavior occurs so that parents can be prepared; primary care giver should ask grandparents, friends, & spouse to spend more time with infant while s/he is present. Touching & cuddling nourish the infant & toddler. Games such as "peek-a-boo" & "all gone" with toys may begin awareness of loss and adjustment to loss.

— Observe behaviors & listen attentively to toddler; be matter of fact & honest, "Grandpa can't come to dinner because he's dead & in (heaven, cemetary or other explanation)." Let toddler have ritual sameness & state that dead person will return only in thoughts & memories. Use correct terms "death," "died," "buried" to prevent confusion; do not use "sleep" to describe death as toddler will be afraid to sleep.

— See NCPG #3:20, "The Child Experiencing Separation Anxiety."

— Know that toddlers are adept at sensing inconsistencies between verbal & non-verbal messages; withholding real feelings will make toddler anxious. Say, "Crying makes me feel better when I'm sad," or "Grownups need to cry & be sad too."

— Teach parents to utilize neighborhood situations to talk about death, i.e., talk about dead birds, bugs, autumn leaves, or dead flowers; read age-appropriate books (see Recommended References) & let child draw pictures; refer to NCPG #3:30, "Play Therapy." Attachment to pets with loss of pet to death is

Believes that thought is sufficient to cause events; this "magical thinking" leads to guilt, shame, and self-punishment. May resent sibling or same-sex parent and wish them dead; if the person then dies, child feels responsible for death.

May giggle, joke, or regress to earlier developmental skills from threat of loss or death; may act as if nothing has happened or may be angry at dead person for abandoning him/her.

3) **Five to nine year old:** conceptualizes death in a concrete sense, as a person such as the "boogy-man," an angel, or a dead person. Is aware that death is permanent but unaware that s/he will die.

Behaviors of beginning awareness that self or loved ones will die include: sleep disturbances, wanting to be with parents at night, preoccupation, and crying. Child may have many questions about death, what happens to dead people, what death feels like.

Fears mutilation and punishment associated with death. May seek out scary stories, movies, games and then have nightmares.

important experience to prepare child for loss of significant person. Allow child to have funeral ritual for pet; don't be surprised if curious child digs up the remains to see if still in ground. Explain in terms child can understand, e.g., "Dead people (animals) cannot eat or run or play or be sad or happy."

— Tell pre-schooler that people cannot be "wished away," inform child that everyone has these wishes sometimes & that thoughts & wishes cannot hurt others. Know that pre-schoolers accept literal meaning of words; listen to thoughts & feelings & clarify understanding of death.

— Accept expressed feelings; give support until child feels safe enough & has enough self-control to grieve & begin to resolve loss. Know that holding & touching comforts pre-schooler. Say "It's OK to cry (or be angry);" let child know that s/he was not at fault or responsible for death.

— Assess understanding & clarify meanings of statements & questions; ask "What do you think makes people (animals) die?" This age group responds well to logical explanation.

— Be willing to listen to religious orientation & beliefs; allow child to talk about feelings; provide aggressive outlets through play, as well as opportunities to draw, write, read & tell stories. Use physical contact & bedtime rituals to encourage to talk about the happenings of the day—joys, fears, concerns, questions. Talking to friends & older siblings may be comforting or scary.

May show much interest in death of relatives or may seem unconcerned.

May worry about who would care for him/her if parents died.

4) **Nine through adolescence:** Begin to be aware that death is inevitable and permanent; see death as far in the future. Know that loved ones and self will die "someday". Mature realization depends upon maturity of child or adolescent.
Adolescents act as if they were invincible — i.e., "Nothing can happen to me," and "Safety rules were made for other people and don't apply to me." — yet they are vulnerable with thoughts of death and concern for possible loss of self, identity, and future. Suicide is an increasing problem in adolescents.
May dramtize and over-react to death of loved one or friend, or may withdraw and not talk about feelings.

— Allow child to attend funeral & burial services; prepare by telling what to expect in matter-of-fact way. Arrange for a friend or family member to sit with child & take child out of service if child wants to leave. Take child to burial site to visit relative's grave if child desires. Answer questions about post-death activities (mortuary, autopsy or funerals).

— Know that support given to parents about their concerns & feelings about death will help child. Allow child to laugh & play during periods of bereavement; play is the work of the child & will facilitate grief work.

— Acknowledge child's concerns & fears about parents, possible death; let child know that they are not dying, & if they did, who would care for the child.

— Know that children mature earlier today than 25 years ago & many have mature concepts of death at 9-12 years. Listen to thoughts & feelings about death; answer questions honestly; discuss movies, television, & books with theme of death.

— Treat adolescent with respect & as an individual who needs guidance & support & need to retain independence, control & decision-making power. Know that peer relationships, rules, & beliefs are important; facilitate peer-group contact.

— Accept expressed feelings of anger or resentment; assist family to regard unpredictable outbursts or projection of anger toward staff or parents as normal response to grief & mourning; observe for misconceptions & leftover "magical thinking" or responsibility/guilt for death. Focus on normalcy of experimentation with independence, sexuality, & aggression so that adolescent will let go of inappropriate guilt. Listen & give support to parents so that they can support adolescent & believe in his/her growing process as mature person.

Recommended References

"Attitudes Towards Death Education for Young Children," by D.R. Crase. *Death Education*, Spring 1979:31-40.

"Books to Help Children Understand Death," by G.G. Mills. *The American Journal of Nursing*, February 1979:291-295.

"The Child & Death," by L.C. Pugh. *Issues in Mental Health Nursing*, December 1979:53-65.

"The Child Experiencing Separation Anxiety." *NCP Guide #3:20*, Nurseco, 1977.

"The Development of a Child's Concept of Death," by S. Johnson-Soderberg. *Oncology Nursing Forum*, Winter 1981:23-26.

"The Parent Experiencing Grief & Loss." *NCP Guide #3:29*, Nurseco, 1977.

"Play Therapy: General Suggestions." *NCP Guide #3:30*, Nurseco, 1977.

"Responses to Loss: The Grief & Mourning Process." *NCP Guide #1:31*, 2nd Ed., Nurseco, 1980.

"Sibling Counseling," by S. Everson. *The American Journal of Nursing*, April 1976:644.

Books for Children: (from The Shanti Project, 1137 Colusa Avenue, Berkeley, CA 94707)

The Accident by C. Carrick. New York: Seabury, 1976 (recommended ages 2-10).

Annie and the Old One by Miska Miles. Boston: Little, Brown, 1971 (ages 8-10 years).

Day by Day by Ron Shuman. Oakland, CA: Scrimshaw, 1977 (8 and over).

First Snow by Helen Coutant. New York: Knopf, 1974 (ages 8-10 years).

Learning to Say Goodbye, by Eda LeShan. New York: Macmillan, 1976 (8 and over).

The Magic Moth by Virginia Lee. New York: Seabury, 1972 (11 and over).

The Tenth Good Thing about Barney by Judith Viorst. New York: Atheneum, 1971 (ages 2-7 years).

The Child with Gastroenteritis

Definition: Acute infectious gastroenteritis is an inflammation of the stomach and intestinal tract caused by pathogenic microorganisms.

LONG TERM GOAL: The child has restored normal gastrointestinal function and motility essential to continuing growth and well-being; the child suffers no after-effects of temporary dehydration and electrolyte imbalance.

General Considerations:
— **Signs & symptoms:** vomiting, diarrhea, lethargy, anorexia, fever, oliguria, and weight loss. Depending on the age and weight of the child and the duration and severity of symptoms, dehydration and electrolyte imbalance may occur fairly rapidly: 24 hours for infants under 3 months and less than 48 hours for babies up to a year.
— A physical examination, along with hematocrit and serum electrolyte studies, defines the state of dehydration and electrolyte imbalance.
— Infants and toddlers are the most vulnerable to gastroenteritis infections and have the poorest compensatory mechanisms to counteract dehydration, electrolyte disturbances, and pathogenic invaders. This is because the water weight of infants comprises 75-80% of their body weight compared to an adult's 60% water/body weight. Also compared with adults, infants, and small children have a greater percentage of extra-cellular water (more easily lost), more body surface in relation to weight, more immature kidney function (less ability to conserve water), greater metabolic rate and greater water turnover rate.
— **Treatment aims:** to control symptoms; to replace and maintain fluids and electrolytes; and to remove, if possible, causative pathogenic organisms.
— **Nursing responsibilities** include the planning, implementation, and evaluation of treatment plan, on-going assessment of hydration/electrolyte status, education of the parent/guardian regarding resumption of care at home, and prevention of further gastroenteritis episodes.
— For further information review the following: NCPGs #3:22-26, "Normal Growth and Development: Newborn to Adolescent;" #3:17, "The Child with Diarrhea;" #3:49, #49, "Fluids & Electrolytes: Parts A & B;" #2:46, "Intravenous Therapy: General Principles;" #3:43, "Diets: Diarrhea Control:" and #3:32, "Teaching the Parent/Guardian/Child: General Suggestions."

Specific Considerations, Potential Patient Outcomes, and Nursing Actions:

1) Control of Symptoms, Provision of Comfort and Security

The child experiences a cessation of vomiting, a reduction in fever, a lessening number of loose, watery stools and a relief of abdominal cramping; the child is comfortable:
  - observe, assess, & record signs & symptoms on admission as well as on an ongoing basis;
  - monitor vital signs; weigh regularly as scheduled; record I&O carefully;
  - maintain NPO until/unless otherwise ordered (to place GI tract at rest);
  - administer prescribed medications (sedatives, antidiarrheics, antibiotics) as ordered; record response to treatment;
  - keep child as clean, dry, & comfortably positioned as possible;
  - provide mouth & lip moistening & lubrication;
  - protect perianal skin with prompt diaper/underpants changes, cleansing, & use of soothing ointments (Note: do not use hydrocortisone cream if using plastic pants, as absorption with resulting side effects is enhanced.);
  - meet the need for oral or sucking satisfaction in the young infant & child with a pacifier or teething toy; burp baby PRN to expel swallowed air;
  - change position at least Q2H & hold babies & small children to minimize crying (it adds to swallowed air & abdominal distention) & to provide comfort.

2) Fluid & Electrolyte Maintenance

The child has good skin turgor, moist mucous membranes, and normal gastrointestinal function — retaining food and fluid; the child regains a normal fluid and electrolyte balance and has nutritional requirements met:
  - monitor for signs of increasing dehydration (less elastic skin turgor, depressed fontanels, sunken eyes, weight loss, rapid pulse, decreasing urine output); chart & report to Dr.;
  - monitor IV hourly; regulate fluids through a microdrop chamber, altering rate as Dr.'s orders change; protect venipuncture site with plastic cup or commercial device; restrain pt. PRN to maintain IV patency; check restraints Q1H for pressure & position;
  - reduce insensible fluid loss (via skin & lungs) by decreasing temp. elevations with tepid sponge baths, meds. as ordered & minimal clothing;
  - follow lab. reports daily & compare them with pt.'s clinical appearance to verify response;

            — when oral fluids are permitted, resume gradually using sterile water or electrolyte solution; progress from half-strength formula to full strength; depending on causative agent, previous diets &/or food preparation habits may need to be changed, so assess & plan accordingly; toleration of new diet or reappearance of vomiting or diarrhea must be promptly & accurately reported; refer to NCPG #3:43, "Diets: Diarrhea Control."

3) Isolation &   The patient's infectious organism causing gastroenteritis is identified and controlled; the patient is free of
    Removal of   secondary infections; the patient is free of emotional and sensory disturbance related to isolation status:
    Causative   — keep pt. isolated from other children & visitors; refer to your hospital procedure;
    Agent   — use strict handwashing techniques when handling pt., diapers, or bedding;
                   — double bag and/or soak all linens & materials leaving room to prevent spread of organism;
                   — interview for possible causes; arrange for communicable disease reporting procedures PRN;
                   — prepare carefully &/or sterilize all formula & fluids given to pt.;
                   — observe pt. hourly to check IV, vital signs, & sensorium; take time for physical & verbal contact;
                   — during acute phase, if ordered, test all stools for blood, sugar & protein; send specimens to lab. for analysis;
                   — instruct parents in the proper method of making, storing & giving formula & meals; reinforce with facts & examples of good handwashing technique & sanitation habits; have parents do a return demonstration (include sitters, older siblings PRN);
                   — teach parents & care-takers early symptoms of illness along with importance & need for prompt medical attention;
                   — encourage parents to visit and interact with pt. to reduce sensory deprivation caused by isolation; use washable or disposable toys, pictures & mobiles that are bright & colorful to stimulate & vary environment; provide musical background when nurse or parents are not in room.

Discharge Planning and Teaching Objectives/Outcomes
1) (Parents/Guardian) Can state how to prevent a recurrence, can identify relevant causes and implement a remedy.
2) Recognize danger signs of vomiting and diarrhea (more than three episodes within a four hour period, loss of appetite, inability to retain fluids or food, fever, change in breathing, diminished urination) along with the need for prompt medical care.

3) Will try to keep child away from sources of infection whenever possible.

4) Say they understand the need to keep child well hydrated, especially in illness.

Recommended References

"Diets: Diarrhea Control." *NCP Guide #3:43*, Nurseco, 1977.

"Fluids & Electrolytes: Parts A & B." *NCP Guides #3:48, 49*, Nurseco, 1977.

"Intravenous Therapy: General Principles." *NCP Guide #2:46*, 2nd Ed., Nurseco, 1980.

"Normal Growth & Development: Newborn to Adolescent." *NCP Guides #3:20-26*, Nurseco, 1977.

"Teaching the Parent/Guardian/Child: General Suggestions." *NCP Guide #3:32*, Nurseco, 1977.

The Child with Sickle Cell Anemia

Definition: Sickle cell anemia is a severe, chronic, inherited disorder of hemoglobin.

LONG TERM GOAL: The child will live as long as possible with minimum necessary limitations and restrictions; the family will support the child and accept limitations placed on the child as s/he grows and develops; the family will adjust to the potential loss of the child.

General Considerations:
— **Incidence:** Usually a disease of black people, one of every 400 black babies has sickle cell anemia; one in every 10 black Americans carries the sickle cell trait.
— **Prognosis:** Decreases life expectancy but childhood death is not universal and should not be considered to be the fate of the child. The cause of death is usually an overwhelming infection or congestive heart failure, and often occurs before 20 years of age. There is no known cure.
— **Clinical course:** *Sickling* results when the O_2 in the hemoglobin drops and the red blood cells are forced into an elongated sickle-like shape. *Sickle cell crisis* occurs when sickled cells pile up against one another in small blood vessels, causing ischemia and infarction in nearby organs and tissues with symptoms of swelling and severe pain; it may be precipitated by infection, fever, increased activity, extreme cold, increased altitude, or trauma resulting in bruising. Clinical problems usually
— arise between six months and two years of age.
Types of sickle cell pathology:
  1) *Sickle cell disease:* active sickling occurs. Two parents with the disease transmit it to *all* offspring; if one parent has the disease, the children have a 50% chance of having the disease and a 50% chance of being carriers of the trait.
  2) *Sickle cell trait:* no active sickling disease, but the trait is inherited from parents and passed on to children. If both parents have the trait, each child has a 25% chance of having sickle cell disease, a 25% chance of being without the disease or trait, and a 50% chance of being a carrier. There is no effect on mortality.
  3) Other types include: *sickle C disease,* an active sickling that is less severe than sickle cell disease. It is inherited when one parent has sickle cell disease and one has hemoglobin C disease; most people affected live to adulthood. *Sickle thalassemia* is caused by inheriting sickle cell disease from one parent and thalassemia from another; symptoms are similar to sickle cell anemia, and may range from mild to severe.

- **Signs and symptoms:** Greyish skin, conjunctiva, and mucous membranes; dyspnea, lethargy, leg ulcers, puffy hands and feet (dactylitis), limping, extreme pain in extremities, joints, abdominal organs.
- **Treatment:** Symptomatic and supportive and may include: transfusions, intravenous fluids, preventing and treating infection, pain control measures, parent and child education, genetic counseling, and emotional support.
- **Nursing responsibilities** include measures for symptom control, providing activities and limits depending on the age and ability of the child, teaching parents and child about the disease, and offering emotional support.

Specific Considerations, Potential Patient Outcomes, and Nursing Actions:

1) Adjustment to Diagnosis of Sickle Cell Disease

The parents and child work through stages of loss; the parents work through grief and mourning about passing on disease to child, and know the genetic consequences of the disease:
- assess parents for current stage of loss & coping (see NCPG #1:31, "Responses to Loss"); encourage them to talk about their feelings & fears by setting aside private time to focus & listen to concerns & feelings (see NCPG #3:29, "The Parent Experiencing Grief and Loss");
- observe for guilt feelings & reinforce clearly that the parents are *not* to blame;
- refer parents to genetic counseling or for contraceptive information as needed; parents need to be aware of risk of having other children with trait or disease;
- spend time listening to child & offer opportunity to express feelings & concerns about illness; explain what is happening to him in terms that s/he can understand; use role playing & play therapy to explore feelings & to health teach; teach parents to assess for fear & anxiety & to practice using role playing as a way to alleviate child's fears & anxieties; refer to NCPG #3:30, "Play Therapy;"
- discuss positive aspects of the disease & life experiences child is able to have; know that sickle cell disease does not affect intelligence; between episodes of crisis, child can participate in school & social life.

2) Treatment During Crisis

The child experiences relief of pain and noxious symptoms; the child receives treatment and emotional support during crisis:
- assess frequently for pain; offer pain medication & heat to area as ordered; know that this type of pain is intense;
- position for comfort; turn often, & give back & skin care; provide mouth care before & after meals; assess child's preferred fluids & offer frequently; record I&O;
- maintain intravenous therapy, including blood transfusions, as ordered;
- know that leg ulcers are common; if present, keep clean & free from infection;

— assist child to plan day so that activity periods are followed by rest periods; plan treatments & activities of daily living around rest periods;

— encourage parents to bring child's books, games, homework, radio or tape recorder to hospital; use these activities to help the child focus on his healthy part & away from his pain & discomfort; assist child to stay in touch with friends by telephone, letters, & visiting;

— assess feelings & concerns of child & parents; offer self as active listener; accept feelings & give support; let child know it is all right to be angry, sad, depressed, just as it is all right to be happy.

3) **Prevention of Crisis**

Parents and older child verbalize contributing factors to sickle cell crisis; parents and older child adapt life style to include crisis-prevention measures:

— assess knowledge of prevention of crisis; teach to avoid exposure to extreme cold, persons with infection, exercise beyond endurance, rough housing or any activity resulting in trauma or bruising, & high altitudes; stress importance of pacing self according to stamina limitations;

— discuss signs of infection that should be reported immediately (lethargy, pallor, fever);

— offer well-balanced diet with meat, green leafy vegetables & fresh fruit, plenty of fluids;

— health teach child & parents to facilitate adjustment to sickling as a chronic illness that needs life-long therapy & medical attention; refer to NCPG #5:30, "The Patient Adjusting to Chronic Illness."

4) **Raising a Child with Sickling**

The parents supply love and set limits needed by child without overprotecting; the child experiences growth and development to reach own potential within limits of chronic illness:

— encourage activities & skills within the child's growth & development status (see NCPGs #3:22-26, "Normal Growth & Development;" mental development is usually unaffected & hobbies & schoolwork are important to the child;

— know & teach parents that child may develop slower than unaffected child & may grow slower & weigh less than his peers;

— be aware, & teach parents, that rules & limits are needed; tyranny by the sick child is to be avoided; parents need to discuss treatment plan with siblings & extended family; encourage family to set limits & not overprotect child; other children in the family need attention & limits as well; teach parents not to give all their attention to sick child.

5) **Raising the Adolescent with Sickling** The parents understand that the sickle cell adolescent has the same developmental needs as the non-sickling adolescent; the adolescent has his needs for peer group knowledge, sex education, birth control, and independence met:

— encourage adolescent to talk about concerns & feelings re: developing body; teenagers & adults with sickle cell anemia have a "spider body" stature with narrow shoulders & hips, kyphosis of upper & lower back, a tower-shaped skull, & an increase in anterior-posterior diameter of the chest; see NCPG #2:29, "The Patient Experiencing a Body Image Disturbance;"

— encourage parents to let the adolescent do as much for himself as possible to facilitate independence, & to trust the adolescent's ability to assume responsibility for himself in a gradual way; reinforce that the adolescent needs involvement with peer group & independence;

— assess adolescent's need for sex & birth control information, & health teach as needed; pregnancy is dangerous for the developing female adolescent with sickling & should be avoided; explain to both sexes the chance of passing on the disease to offspring; refer for genetic counseling or birth control as desired & needed; encourage any questions the adolescent has about dating, sex, or birth control;

— assess the need for vocational counseling & make referrals PRN.

6) **Psychosocial Adjustment to Potential Loss** The child and parents deal adaptively with the illness of the child in crisis and the child who is terminal; the child is supported physically and emotionally:

— refer to NCPGs #1:27, "Impending Death," #1:31, "Responses to Loss," #4:25, "The Child who is Dying/Terminal," & #5:24, "The Child's Conception of Death;"

— assess child & family members for stage of grieving & behavioral responses; support adaptive responses & offer self as caring, interested listener; remember that the family has been dealing with a chronic illness for a long time;

— spend time with pt. & family, encouraging them to express their feelings & to grieve openly; know that your presence is comforting to them; refer to NCPG #5:45, "Hospice Care Concepts;"

— provide comfort measures for both pt. & family; accept them in their time of loss & grief.

Discharge Planning and Teaching Objectives/Outcomes

1) (Patient/Family/Significant Other) Has an appointment for follow up with physician or clinic, and can state the importance of keeping all appointments even when symptom-free.

2) Knows factors that contribute to sickle cell crisis and to avoid or minimize them in life style as much as possible; knows to contact physician or clinic at first signs of pallor, jaundice, lethargy, fever, or pain.

3) States importance of regular immunizations and immunization against pneumococcus.

4) Has needed referrals for counseling (genetic, sex education, birth control, support groups).

Recommended References

"The Child who is Dying/Terminal." *NCP Guide #4:25*, Nurseco, 1978.

"The Child's Conception of Death." *NCP Guide #5:24*, Nurseco, 1981.

"Home Management of Sickle Cell Anemia," by Carol Flanagan. *Pediatric Nurse*, March-April 1980: B-D.

"Hospice Care Concepts." *NCP Guide #5:45*, Nurseco, 1981.

"Normal Growth & Development: Newborn, Infant, Toddler/Preschool, School Age Child, Adolescent." *NCP Guides #s 3:22-26*, Nurseco, 1977.

"The Parent Experiencing Grief and Loss." *NCP Guide #3:29*, Nurseco, 1977.

"The Patient Experiencing a Body Image Disturbance." *NCP Guide #2:29*, Nurseco, 1980.

"The Patient Adapting to Chronic Illness Role." *NCP Guide #5:30,* Nurseco, 1981.

"Play Therapy: General Suggestions." *NCP Guide #3:30,* Nurseco, 1977.

"Responses to Loss: The Grief and Mourning Process." *NCP Guide #1:31*, 2nd Ed., Nurseco, 1980.

"Sickle Cell Anemia: Current Concepts," by Carl A. Reindorf. *Pediatric Nurse*, March-April 1980: E-G.

"Sickle Cell Disorders," by J. McFarland. *The American Journal of Nursing*, December 1977: 1948-1954.

The Diabetic Postpartum Patient

LONG TERM GOAL: The diabetic postpartum patient will experience a safe, satisfying outcome for herself and baby; she will assume parental role and responsibilities with satisfaction and a minimum of tolerable tension; she will complete the bio-psycho-social process of involution and restoration without preventable complications; she will regain pre-pregnancy control of her diabetes.

General Considerations:
— For the diabetic patient, whether delivery is by caesarian section or induced vaginal method, the fourth stage of labor is a time of intensive care to prevent complications, primarily of toxemia, hemorrhage, infection, and hypoglycemia. Control of diabetes and bio-psycho-social stabilization are the aims of medical and nursing care.

— The postpartum period (at least 6 weeks after delivery) is a vulnerable period of recovery and stabilization for the family (mother, father, infant, siblings, and grandparents). Rapid physical, psychological, and emotional changes in a very short time span are energy draining and produce a "future shock" situation abundant with strained relationships, negative feelings, and role disturbances even in the most "normal" and healthy family. For the diabetic mother there is heightened concern for the health of her newborn who may be receiving neonatal intensive care and be hospitalized for several weeks after she has gone home. Follow-up home visits by the community health nurse are valuable in assisting the family to cope with the necessary adjustments. If she delivered a stillborn, there will be enormous problems coping with the grief and loss in light of the risks and care the mother has taken to have a healthy infant; see NCPG #3:29, "The Parent Experiencing Grief & Loss."

— **Nursing responsibilities** are to:
  (1) support the bio-psycho-social process of involution and recovery, thus preventing complications and providing comfort;

(2) assist the patient to return to pre-pregnancy diet, insulin, and control of diabetes;
(3) counsel the patient regarding appropriate birth control methods;
(4) help the parents internalize the reality of their labor and delivery experience in order to proceed toward successful parent/child attachment;
(5) facilitate a harmonious family integration and adaptation that will be mutually supportive in the months ahead; and
(6) arrange for home nursing referral and follow-up medical care for both mother and child.

— If the patient has had a caesarian section, nursing responsibilities proceed from a view of the mother as a post-op abdominal patient, a postpartum patient, and a diabetic. See NCPG #4:31, "The Mother with a Caesarian Section Birth," as well as the nursing guides on diabetes listed in the Recommended References.

Specific Considerations, Potential Patient Outcomes, and Nursing Actions:

1) Prevention of Complic-ations
The patient has a normally contracted uterus and normal lochia; the patient has a healing perineum; the patient gives own perineal care and insulin injections as soon as able; the patient is afebrile, free of infection, hemorrhage, toxemia, hypertension, hypoglycemia, and acidosis; otherwise, these complications are promptly detected and adequately controlled:

— check vital signs, post recovery room, at least Q4H for 48 hours; report promptly BP increases;
— be sure that blood sugar was drawn while pt. was in recovery room, or have it done as soon as possible;
— check urine for S&A Q2H & maintain accurate records; have pt. do this as soon as able;
— monitor IV fluids at prescribed rate; maintain accurate I&O records;
— observe pt. for signs of hyper- & hypoglycemia; see NCPG #1:35, "Differentiating Hypoglycernia & Ketoacidosis,"
— adjust insulin as prescribed, keeping in mind serum & urine glucose levels as well as pt.'s intake; let pt. take over insulin injections when she is able;
— check level & firmness of fundus Q30min. x 4, Q1H x 4, then Q6H & PRN; know that uterine atony caused by excessive amniotic fluid is a common cause of hemorrhage & that oxytocin is often prescribed;
— check perineum, hemorrhoids, & episiotomy QID for bright red bleeding; note & record no. of saturated perineal pads per 8 hrs;

— observe & record color, odor, & amt. of lochia QID;
— assist pt. to provide own perineal care when able, including hand washing before & after care, warm, sterile water cleansing after elimination, daily shower with antibacterial soap, thorough drying, heat lamp 15-20 min. TID, palliative spray if ordered, aseptic application of clean perineal pad; sitz baths QID may be desirable for acute discomfort;
— observe for post saddle/spinal anesthesia headaches & report if present; keep pt. flat in bed without pillow, force fluids, apply abdominal binder & give PRN analgesic.

2) Breast Care   The patient experiences lactation (or its suppression if not breast-feeding) with a minimum of tolerable discomfort; the patient has no preventable complications (or they are promptly identified and correctly managed):
— *if not nursing,* apply breast binder or snug fitting bra; use ice packs to each breast at least 3-4 times daily & give aspirin or other prescribed analgesic for breast discomfort; do not pump breasts; give med. to suppress lactation;
— *if nursing,* wash nipples with warm water to remove dried, oozing colostrum PRN, to prevent dryness & cracking, use no soap or irritant; apply Vit. A&D Ointment or nipple cream after nursing to provide lubrication; have pt. change breast pads frequently;
— know that breast-feeding is not contraindicated because insulin does not enter milk; refer PRN to NCPG #4:30, "The Mother who Breast-feeds Her Infant;"
— know that a diabetic pt. is particularly susceptible to infections of all kinds; teach pt. to observe & report cracks, irritation, redness, warmth, tenderness of her breasts & fever of 37.50°C. (99.5°F.); if present, mother should discontinue nursing, manually express milk, & call Dr.;
— teach pt. that, for engorged breasts, a degree of relief can be obtained with warm, moist compresses for 20 min. &/or by expressing milk by hand or by pump methods.

| 3) Maintenance of Normal Body Functions Nutrition, Elimination, Exercise, Rest/Sleep | The patient tolerates prescribed ADA diet; the patient re-establishes a normal pattern of elimination (voiding QS and normal stool); the patient ambulates as desired; the patient sleeps for 3-6 hrs. at a time and says she feels rested: |

- when IVs are discontinued, liquids & soft foods will probably be introduced sometime during postpartal day one; note & record tolerance & intake; refer to NCPG #1:37, "Diabetes: Liquid Diet Substitutes;"
- if mother is breast-feeding, diet & insulin will have to be modified accordingly; know that her diet should be increased at least 400 calories a day. of which at least one-fourth should be additional protein; be sure pt. understands that when she decides to wean her infant — or should she have to stop nursing suddenly for some reason — she needs to inform her physician so diet & insulin can be adjusted accordingly;
- give ADA diet as tolerated & ordered; have snacks available, so that pt. can treat any signs of hypoglycemia that are likely to occur as the catabolic process of involution takes place & lowers blood sugar;
- check voiding (amt., frequency, & appearance); be alert for bladder distention or residual retention;
- check bowel movements; give suppository, laxative, or enema as ordered & needed; teach pt. to wipe in a backward direction from vagina, using facial or very soft toilet tissue;
- help pt. to get up to bathroom & chair first time after delivery; ambulate as desired after first 4-6 hours post delivery; be sure abdominal binder is snugly in place; check pt.'s BP before & after getting up;
- encourage walking before naps & night time sleep; help pt. to relax with reading, relaxation exercises & controlled breathing, or visual imagery techniques; see NCPG #5:49, "Stress Management;"
- give PRN med. for discomfort & for sleep (unless contraindicated because of breast-feeding);
- try to avoid disturbing pt. so needs for rest can be adequately met; inquire how pt. feels after sleep & record response; know that sleep deprivation & emotional tension of postpartum period can drain energy needed for recovery & resumption of roles;
- discuss with pt. feelings about postpartum figure, expectations, plans for exercise; with Dr. approval, give list of postpartum exercises (see NCPG #3:31); review them with pt. & demonstrate.

4) Psychosocial
   Adjustment
   (to Role
   Change,
   Parenting
   Respons-
   ibilities,
   Postpartum
   Recovery)
   Parent/Infant
   Bonding

The mother (& father) express pleasure in their accomplishment of successful labor with delivery of a live infant (or the parents begin the grief process over the loss of their newborn or birth of a malformed infant); the parents indicate acceptance & understanding of their role and responsibilities as parents by expressing realistic plans for mother and infant care during the first four to six weeks following discharge; the parents display behaviors indicating attachment to their infant:

— encourage parents to verbalize their feelings about labor, delivery, present condition of mother & infant; ask them to re-live & recount their experience;

— keep parents informed of status of infant & mother's condition; answer questions; provide reassurance & hope if this is realistic; assure them the child is normal (if you are certain this is true) & explain what to expect in the way of growth & behavior, if this is a first child; know that infant will not necessarily have diabetes during his lifetime & chances are small that s/he will have the disease as a child;

— if the parents had a stillborn or a malformed infant, see NCPG #3:29, "The Parent Experiencing Grief & Loss;"

— accompany parents to neonatal intensive care unit & observe their visit with baby; consult with neonatal intensive care nurses; assess parent's adaptation to infant: do they have a name for it & call it by name? do they handle baby in a warm, cuddling manner, establishing eye contact? do they speak to baby? what is the feeling tone, manner? do they express pleasure in having baby & in caring for him? if mother and/or father appear tense, look away from baby, cry, keep asking if baby is all right or keep finding negative aspects about infant, explore reasons for their behavior; ask if they could share their feelings with you; if you feel unable to listen or accept this behavior, seek consultation with a parent/child nursing specialist or psychiatric/mental health nursing specialist;

— ask parents how they feel about baby after they have seen it; allow them to ventilate any disappointment over sex, appearance, etc.; refrain from saying, "You should be thankful this baby is alive, considering all you've been through," or any other negative admonishments; ask them about their expectations, dreams re: new child compare this with reality & provide realistic feedback;

— explain natural molding of head, helpfulness of rotating positions (side-to side, prone, & supine) & when to expect closure of fontanels; arrange with mother to attend postpartum baby care classes;

— refer to NCPG #4:32, "Parent-Infant Bonding (Attachment)" for additional information & nursing actions;
— know that mothers of premature infants & infants with congenital abnormalities may need more help & take longer in their attachment process;
— discuss with both parents the phenomenon of "baby blues" or postpartum depression; find out what is known, believed, felt about this; explain that fatigue is a significant & influencing factor & discuss what plans have been made to prevent or relieve fatigue;
— inquire re: the direct (physical) & moral support systems available to parents for the first six weeks after discharge; what professional help is accessible?
— consider if a referral to a community health nurse is desirable to help make arrangements for the infant who probably will be kept at the hospital for a few weeks longer than the mother;
— know that contraceptive information & advice is an important aspect of pt. care, since each successive pregnancy causes more risk to mother & fetus; know & teach pt. that oral contraceptives alter carbohydrate metabolism in a diabetogenic way necessitating more insulin; refer to NCPGs #5:38, "Birth Control: Permanent Methods," & #5:39, "Birth Control: Temporary Methods."

Discharge Planning and Teaching Objectives/Outcomes

1) (Patient/Family/Significant Other) Has written instructions re: diet, exercise, care of perineum & breasts, medications (name, purpose, dosage, side effects, etc.), birth control, and sexual relations; says she understands instructions and intends to comply.
2) Has participated in baby care classes or has indicated she is knowledgeable and confident re: bathing, diapering, feeding and essentials of newborn care (cord stump, circumcision, formula preparation, prevention of illness and injury); has at least one or two infant care books for reference.
3) Has the name and phone number of a health care professional (physician, community health nurse) to call upon for assistance and guidance as desired and needed.
4) Has postpartum check-up appointment slip (date, time, place) and a referral for community health nursing visits PRN.
5) Has an awareness of the infant attachment process and can describe how she will further the process if she is to be separated from her infant until its hospital release.

Recommended References

"Birth Control: Permanent Methods." *NCP Guide #5:38,* Nurseco, 1981.

"Birth Control: Temporary Methods." *NCP Guide #5:39,* Nurseco, 1981.

"Diabetes: Differentiating Hypoglycemia and Ketoacidosis." *NCP Guide #1:35,* 2nd Ed., Nurseco, 1980.

"Diabetes: Liquid Diet Sustitutes." *NCP Guide #1:37,* 2nd Ed., Nurseco, 1980.

"The Mother who Breast-feeds Her Infant." *NCP Guide #4:30,* Nurseco, 1978.

"The Mother with a Caesarian Section Birth." *NCP Guide #1:31,* Nurseco, 1978.

"The Parent Experiencing Grief & Loss." *NCP Guide #3:29,* Nurseco, 1977.

"Parent-Infant Bonding (Attachment)." *NCP Guide #4:32,* Nurseco, 1978.

"Postpartum Exercises." *NCP Guide #3:31,* Nurseco, 1977.

"Stress Management." *NCP Guide #5:49,* Nurseco, 1981.

"When A Pregnant Women is Diabetic: Postpartal Care," by Nancy Rancilio. *The American Journal of Nursing,* March 1979:453-456.

The Pregnant Diabetic: Part A — Antepartal Care

LONG TERM GOAL: The pregnant diabetic will experience trust and confidence in the medical team and will participate knowledgeably in health care decisions; the pregnant diabetic will enter labor with hope for a successful outcome and with the preliminary maternal-infant bonding process begun.

General Considerations:
- **Incidence:** one in 300-500 pregnancies is complicated by diabetes mellitus.
- **Complications and risks** depend on the duration of the patient's diabetes and the extent of vascular disease; they include large baby, large placenta, preeclampsia, spontaneous abortion, intrauterine fetal loss, intrapartum fetal loss, or neonatal loss. In addition, the patient is susceptible to hydramnios (excess amniotic fluid), urinary tract infections (UTIs), and increasingly severe diabetes with its usual complications (hypoglycemia, hyperglycemia, retinopathy).
- The pregnant diabetic should be seen, evaluated and cared for — soon after pregnancy is ascertained — by a team of maternal intensive care specialists: an obstetrician experienced in high-risk pregnancies, an OB clinical nurse specialist, a nutritionist, a social worker, and a neonatologist. Weekly clinic visits are scheduled until diabetic condition becomes difficult to control or complications arise; then the patient is hospitalized until a planned delivery, often in the 36-38th week, when fetal maturity warrants survival.
- A comprehensive history includes an assessment of the patient's knowledge and control of her diabetes, diet, medication, and self-care; review and re-teaching are commonly necessary. In addition, the patient needs to understand the changes that pregnancy will cause and the reasons for the intensive treatment program; refer to the nursing care planning guides on diabetes in the Recommended References.
- If the patient has had previous unsuccessful pregnancies with loss of fetus or newborn, she may have unresolved grief and feelings that need to be resolved before she is able to form a healthy attachment to this fetus; refer to NCPG #1:31, "Responses to Loss: The Grief and Mourning Process." Other concerns of the pregnant diabetic include the likelihood of the healthy newborn developing diabetes as a child (1-10%) as well as typical fears related to the pregnant patients's age, marital status, maturity, and independence.
- **Tests** are used to monitor fetal status and to determine its maturity and readiness to survive birth. These should be understood by the nurse and explained to patient and family so that satisfactory cooperation and results can be obtained. Commonly used tests include:

- *Ultrasonography:* a safe, non-invasive means of "seeing" the moving fetus and measuring the biparietal diameter (distance between the two parietal bones of cranium). Polaroid pictures can be taken and given to parents; the mother is encouraged to see and speak to fetus, and a number of fetal structures are pointed out to her by the radiologist. This helps offset the patient's discomfort from the hard examining table, the cold contact gel, and having to have a full bladder for the test.
- *Amniocentesis:* a 22-gauge needle is inserted through the anesthetized skin of the abdomen to obtain 10-20 ml. of amniotic fluid; examination can show genetic abnormalities and sex. To assess maturity of fetal lungs, lab technicians determine the ratio of concentrated lecithin and sphingomyelin. L/S ratios over a minimum 2:1 indicate acceptable lung maturity. Sometimes IM steroids are given to mother to promote fetal lung maturity just prior to planned delivery.
- *Urinary estriol:* placental hormone levels rise with advancing pregnancy; measured in urine, a 50% drop over previous level indicates placental insufficiency. Twenty-four hour urine specimens are collected and examined up to three times weekly from the 30th week on. The patient is given unbreakable, leak-proof bottles; refrigeration is unnecessary.
- *Fetal heart rate tests:* now performed electronically with Doppler transducers, are done weekly from the 28th week on. External monitoring is done until labor has progressed sufficiently to allow internal monitoring with electrodes attached to fetal scalp. Fetal heart rates (FHR) are monitored and graphed during response to the stress of uterine contractions (Oxytocin Challenge Test — OCT) as well as during normal relaxed periods (Nonstress Test — NST). FHR is also studied in relation to fetal movement (Fetal Activity Acceleration Determinations — FAD). The OCT assesses the respiratory function of the placenta. If the FHR shows late decelerations during contractions, it means there is a low respiratory placental reserve and therefore decreased oxygenation to the fetus during a contraction; an adequate reserve shows the fetus can be maintained satisfactorily a week longer. Oxytocin is given via infusion pump to ensure precise control of administration. It is not given if there is sufficient spontaneous uterine activity to provide necessary information on FHR response to contractions.

Specific Considerations, Potential Patient Outcomes, and Nursing Actions:

1) Control of Diabetes

The patient's diabetic control is maintained; the fetus is not exposed to maternal acidosis:
- on scheduled weekly clinic/office visits, monitor & record pt.'s blood sugars & urine S & A;
- explain need to maintain home records of urine S & A QID, & to report immediately three successive 3 + urine sugar levels or a positive acetone; assess response to medications & record;
- assess response to medications & record;

- review signs & symptoms of hyper- & hypoglycemia;
- if pt. has been on oral hypoglycemics, teach insulin administration in preparation for when injections become necessary;
- explain to pt. that, when delivery is imminent, the insulin dose will be reduced to prepare her body to return to pre-pregnancy levels & to reduce risk of neonatal hypoglycemia;
- arrange for dietitian to meet with pt. to plan diet; know that a high protein (2 gm/KgBW), high-CHO, & low-sodium (1 Gm.) daily intake is desired;
- determine adequacy of skin & feet care; health teach PRN;
- for additional nursing actions, refer to NCPGs on diabetes listed in the Recommended References.

2) Progress of Pregnancy

Maternal and fetal status progress according to schedule without complications; maternal infections are prevented or promptly treated:

- record pt.'s weight, BP, TPR each visit, reporting significant increases;
- examine pt.'s extremities for signs of edema; question for headaches, blurred vision, swollen fingers or ankles, & report accordingly;
- examine urinalysis report & query pt. for symptoms of UTI (pain or burning on micturition, itching, fever); urge pt. to drink adequate daily fluids (unless restricted); if UTI exists, ascertain that pt. takes full course of antibiotics as prescribed & returns for a repeat urinalysis;
- observe & query for increasing abdominal or bilateral groin pain; note whether contractions are irregular, widely spaced & non-progressive, or regular with increasing frequency; since premature contractions can prompt labor, request pt. immediately to rest quietly in bed until hospitalization can be arranged; try to allay apprehension by telling pt. that this is a common occurence & doesn't necessarily mean a premature delivery;
- assess pt.'s previous knowledge of fetal monitoring; explain to pt. PRN & assist her to cooperate with various tests to monitor fetal status & maturity; assure pt./family of the safety & reliability of tests as well as the value of information provided; stay with pt. during test providing support, comfort, reassurance, & progress reports; use waiting time to review controlled breathing & relaxation exercises with pt.; be sure pt. is regularly attending prenatal classes (preferably with spouse/significant other or a labor coach substitute);
- know & explain to pt. that delivery is planned for sometime during the 36-38th week of pregnancy, depending on outcome of tests.

3) Psychosocial Adjustment & Maternal-Infant Bonding

The patient's physical and mental activity is sustained at optimum levels; the patient copes adaptively with stresses of a high-risk pregnancy, participating cooperatively in her plan of care; the patient initiates maternal-infant bonding; the patient expresses optimism and confidence for a successful outcome of her pregnancy:
- encourage pt. to make things for baby, learning, if necessary, how to knit, crochet, embroider or do other needlework; suggest other diversional activities & recommend reading material for time spent waiting in hospital or offices;
- encourage pt. to purchase a baby book & begin to make entries; have pt. arrange with family or friend to save newspaper headlines for the day of birth;
- spend time talking with pt. & husband re: concerns, fears, worries; encourage hope, but do not provide false reassurance if risks are enhancing & prognosis is doubtful;
- during fetal monitoring or ultrasound exams, talk to fetus & encourage mother to do so; speculate on sex, if unknown; talk about prospective name choices; provide pt. with Polaroid picture of sonogram showing fetal outline; make a tape recording of fetal heart rate during one of the OCTs so that pt. can share excitement with family & friends;
- for additional nursing actions, refer to NCPG #4:32, "Parent-Infant Bonding."

Discharge Planning and Teaching Objectives/Outcomes

1) (Patient/Family/Significant Other) Understands the changes that pregnancy makes upon diabetes and demonstrates ability and willingness to cooperate with modified prenatal care and diabetes management.
2) Recognizes need to observe and promptly report all untoward signs of impending complications; has a written list of instructions.
3) Demonstrates confidence in a successful outcome and makes realistic arrangements for baby room, clothing, care, etc.).
4) Makes provisions for unexpected emergency hospitalizations should they be necessary, and plans for an early hospitalization approximately four weeks before due date.
5) Has social service referral, if needed, for homemaker services or financial assistance and has a community health nursing referral for home care visits.

Recommended References

"Corinne: A Mother at Risk," by Mecca Cranley. *The American Journal of Nursing*, December 1978:2117-2120.

"Diabetes: Differentiating Hypoglycemia and Ketoacidosis." *NCP Guide #1:35*, 2nd Ed., Nurseco, 1980.

"Diabetes: General Dietary Principles." *NCP Guide #1:36*, 2nd Ed., Nurseco, 1980.

"Diabetes: Liquid Diet Substitutes." *NCP Guide #1:37*, 2nd Ed., Nurseco, 1980.

"Diabetes in Pregnancy," by Jane Snyder et al. *Nursing 80*, November 1980:44-49.

"Diabetes: Properties of Insulin Preparations." *NCP Guide #1:38*, 2nd Ed., Nurseco, 1980.

"Diabetes: Recommended Care of the Feet." *NCP Guide #1:39*, 2nd Ed., Nurseco, 1980.

"Oxytocin Challenge Test," by Sarla Sethi. *The American Journal of Nursing*, December 1978:2112 — 2114.

"Parent-Infant Bonding (Attachment)." *NCP Guide #4:32*, Nurseco, 1978.

"Responses To Loss: The Grief and Mourning Process." *NCP Guide #1:31*, 2nd Ed., Nurseco, 1980.

"The Patient with Diabetes." *NCP Guide #1:07*, 2nd Ed., Nurseco, 1980.

"When A Pregnant Woman Is Diabetic: Antepartal Care," by Katherine Schuler. *The American Journal of Nursing*, March 1979:448 — 450.

The Pregnant Diabetic: Part B – Intrapartal Care

LONG TERM GOAL: The pregnant diabetic will experience a safe, comfortable, satisfying delivery of a live infant; she will complete her fourth stage of labor with complications either prevented or promptly and successfully controlled; the mother strengthens the bonding process with her infant with visual, verbal, and physical contact.

General Considerations:
— Review NCPG #5:28, "The Pregnant Diabetic: Part A – Antepartal Care."
— As the pregnant diabetic nears forty weeks gestation, the severity of her diabetes increases, along with the possibility of complications. This makes early, planned delivery desirable. Either an induced labor or caesarian section is expected. The patient is hospitalized from at least the 35th week on, so that maternal and fetal monitoring can determine the course of intensive care needed.
— **Complications of third trimester** include: hyperglycemia, infection (commonly of the urinary tract), hemorrhage, placental dysfunction, preeclampsia, enlarged fetal size with cephalopelvic disproportion.
— **Complications during labor:** hypoglycemia is a problem since glycogen stores are depleted by energy needs, so when delivery is imminent, insulin dosage is reduced and IV infusions of 5 or 10% dextrose in distilled water are given. Induced labor brings dangers of excessive, hard contractions and uterine rupture to mother and possible CNS damage, cord compression, acidosis, FHR (fetal heart rate) deceleration, and hypoxia to newborn. A caesarian section, especially if induced labor has been unsuccessful, brings potential problems of parental anxiety reactions, maternal hypoglycemia, infection, hemorrhage, and delayed abdominal wound healing.
— **Nursing responsibilities** are seriously awesome. Only the most qualified OB nursing clinical specialists should provide the intensive care needed during the crucial intrapartal period for this high-risk patient. Constant conscientious monitoring and assessment, along with prompt, correct intervention are necessary to prevent maternal and fetal complications, to maintain stable physiological systems, and to support psychosocial adaptation in a critical situation.

Specific Considerations, Potential Patient Outcomes, and Nursing Actions:

1) Fluid and Electrolyte Balance

The patient is free of hypo- and hyperglycemia; the patient has sufficient fluid and glucose intake to provide satisfactory (50 ml. minimum) output:
— when ordered, place pt. on NPO & begin IV dextrose in water infusions; maintain accurate flow rate;

- reduce insulin dosage as ordered & explain to pt. that this will reduce risk of hypoglycemia for herself & baby;
- ascertain that blood & urine glucose levels are tested on schedule & recorded promptly; report changes;
- initiate & maintain accurate I&O records;
- check bladder for distention Q2H; observe for pain or burning on micturition, cloudy urine & insufficient output (below 50 ml. minimum/hr.);
- watch for signs of hypoglycemia (tachycardia, hunger, weakness, sweating, tremor, pallor); see NCPG #1:35, "Diabetes: Differentiating Hypoglycemia and Ketoacidosis;" take corrective action (*Note:* hypoglycemia may be related to mother's anxiety; evaluate & intervene for this as well as increase IV rate or percentage of dextrose).

2) Prevention of Compli- cations

The patient and fetus are free of complications, or have them promptly detected and controlled; the patient leaves delivery room in a physiologically stabilized condition or continues with intensive care in recovery room;
- place pt. in semi-Fowler's position to prevent supine hypotension & to promote comfort; tilt her slightly to left side to facilitate utero-placental hemodynamics & an optimum FHR:
- arrange for gown/cap/mask & placement of labor coach assistant; answer questions, provide information, & promote optimism; utilize humor appropriately to reduce tension;
- set up induction & monitoring equipment; be prepared for both external &, later, internal fetal monitoring; explain monitoring equipment & procedures to pt./father/significant other (SO);
- initiate & maintain standard labor records; monitor & record TPR & BP, contractions, oxytocin dosage, cervical dilatation, FHR, etc. as frequently as ordered & needed;
- observe vaginal discharge for excessive bleeding or meconium;
- determine baseline pattern for FHR & variability; observe FHR closely for late & variable deceleration patterns; if occurring, take mother's BP to determine if hypotension is cause; if so, try turning pt. to left side & increase rate of IV infusion; assess whether deceleration is possibly caused by uterine hypertonus; If so, stop oxytocin infusion, start oxygen, & notify obstetrician;
- if caesarian is planned, refer to NCPG #4:31, "The Mother with a Caesarian Section Birth;"
- prepare perineal & abdominal skin areas; administer enema only if specifically ordered as it is often contraindicated; provide for safekeeping of personal belongings.

3) Psychosocial   The patient/father/SO accepts, understands, and cooperates appropriately with the changing situation; the
   Adjustment   patient/father/SO expresses fears and concerns, copes adaptively with stress; the patient/father/SO establishes
   and Bonding   visual, touching, and verbal relationship with infant almost immediately after birth:
   Process   — encourage pt./father/SO to ask questions, express fears & concerns;
                   — take time to provide ongoing explanations of equipment, treatment, safety precautions, & reasons for nursing
                     actions;
                   — share information about pt.'s progress, maintaining optimism & hope;
                   — assist pt. with controlled breathing & relaxation techniques;
                   — help pt. to rest between contractions; provide comfort measures according to pt. wishes; reduce environmental
                     & extraneous stimuli;
                   — arrange for pt./father/SO to see as much of the birth as possible; allow pt./father/SO to see, touch, & speak to
                     newborn; listen to pediatrician's description of newborn condition; provide additional explanations & repeat
                     information PRN to reinforce reality;
                   — refer to NCPG #4:32, "Parent-Infant Bonding (Attachment)," for additional nursing actions & information.

Discharge Planning and Teaching Objectives/Outcomes
Refer to NCPG #5:27, "The Diabetic Postpartum Patient."

Recommended References
"Diabetes: Differentiating Hypoglycemia and Ketoacidosis." *NCP Guide #1:35*, 2nd Ed., Nurseco, 1980.
"Intrapartal Fetal Monitoring." by Marilyn Yumek & Rita Lojex. *The American Journal of Nursing*, December 1978:2102-2109.
"Parent-Infant Bonding (Attachment)." *NCP Guide #4:32*, Nurseco, 1978.
"The Diabetic Postpartum Patient." *NCP Guide #5:27*, Nurseco, 1981.
"The Mother with a Caesarian Section Birth." *NCP Guide #4:31*, Nurseco, 1978.
"The Pregnant Diabetic: Part A — Antepartal Care." *NCP Guide #5:28*, Nurseco, 1981.
"When a Pregnant Woman is Diabetic: Intrapartal Care." by Diane Wimberley. *The American Journal of Nursing*. March 1979:451-452.

The Patient Adapting to Chronic Illness Role

Definition: Chronic illness is considered to be any impairment or deviation from normal health that has some of the following characteristics: 1) permanent, non-reversible, or residual impairment; 2) insidious onset; 3) requires a long period of supervision of care. Chronic illness role consists of behaviors related to the limitations imposed by the impairment or deviation from normal health and behaviors defined by society as appropriate to the limitations.

LONG TERM GOAL: The patient will adapt to limitations imposed by chronic illness; the patient will care for self and be as independent as possible; the patient will be motivated to retain whatever tasks and roles are possible.

General Considerations:
— Chronic illness involves a life-long period of treatment, usually with remissions and exacerbation of symptoms; this role is not seen by society as attractive or desired, and the patient is often separated from the well population during periods of exacerbation.

— Impairment requires special training for rehabilitation; the patient is expected to share in the planning and treatment process and to assume increasing responsibility for self-care.

— **Treatment goal** is to delay or control acute symptoms, promote comfort, maintain healthy bio-psycho-social systems, and rehabilitate to patient's full potential.

— **Nursing assessment** includes assessing the patient for behaviors associated with chronic illness role which may include:

  - hope, hopelessness
  - anger, frustration
  - depression
  - anxiety
  - fear of total disability or death
  - alterations in self-esteem
  - alterations in body-image
  - powerlessness
  - grief and mourning
  - feelings of being stigmatized, shame
  - instrumental and emotional dependence
  - motivation to retain roles and tasks.

— **Nursing responsibilities,** in addition to assessment, are to prevent deformities and complications, to motivate, to teach and support the patient and family in resuming self-care activities, and to refer patient for follow-up care and supervision.

— For additional information, refer to NCPGs #2:29, "Patient Experiencing a Body Image Disturbance," #5:32, "The Patient Experiencing a Threat to Self-Esteem," and #5:34, "The Patient Experiencing Powerlessness."

Specific Considerations, Potential Patient Outcomes, and Nursing Actions:

1) Immediate
   Response to
   Diagnosis of
   Chronic Illness

The patient experiences emotional support while reacting to diagnosis of chronic disease or disability; the patient participates in planning care, does as much self-care as limitations allow, and complies with treatment plan:

— assess pt. for behaviors of shock & disbelief, denial & other behaviors of loss; listen & give emotional support, accepting the pt.'s need to cope with the situation at his own pace; accept pt.'s denial at this time but do not support it (see NCPG #1:24, "The Patient Manifesting Denial");

— protect pt. from injury caused by denying or ignoring limitations; strive to prevent complications & deformities (see NCPGs #2:45, "The Hazards of Immobility" & #1:42, "Effects of Hospitalization: Part C: Prolonged Confinement");

— encourage pt. to participate in planning own care & to do as much self-care as limitations of chronic disease or disability will allow; be aware that pt. may become very dependent on first hearing diagnosis;

— assess pt. & family for knowledge of chronic disease process, treatment plan, treatments, medications, & for feelings & concerns; give positive reinforcement for knowledge & for cooperation with treatment plan;

— offer brief explanations if requested; wait until initial grief & mourning period is over to begin health teaching;

— be aware of adaptive & maladaptive behaviors associated with loss; assess pt.'s behaviors & support adaptive ones; refer to NCPG #1:31, "Responses to Loss;"

— know that pt. is in a state of conflict at forced dependence imposed by limitations with threat to usual lifestyle & self-esteem; maintain hope for rehabilitation without supporting false hopes or unrealistic goals.

2) Adaptation to
   Chronic
   Disease or
   Disability

The patient begins to recognize and cope with limitations; the patient becomes committed to rehabilitation program:

— emphasize pt.'s assets & strengths; give positive reinforcement with praise & attention as pt. begins to show progress & commitment to treatment plan & rehabilitation program;

— set short-term goals with pt. in order to increase ability to be independent in ADL (activities of daily living); encourage pt. to do independent therapeutic exercises & ROM (see NCPG #1:47, "Range of Motion Exercises") as ordered by physician & physical therapist;

— know that participation in ADL & exercise program is essential to restore motivation & optimism in pt., as well as to retain muscle tone & ROM;

— be a creative problem solver with the pt. & the health care team to assist the pt. to use self-help devices when s he has difficulty performing an activity; self-help devices may include adaptive equipment for mobility, personal care aids, communication, writing & typewriting aids (see NCPG #5:47, "Problem Solving");

— assess for readiness to learn about disease process, treatment plan, medication & prognosis; health teach pt. & family as indicated; see NCPGs #1:49 & 50, "Teaching Patients;"

— assess hobbies & pastimes to encourage socialization & to avoid boredom & sensory monotony;

— be aware that persons with chronic illness or disability are still sexual beings; assist pt. to deal with sexual concerns by health teaching, counseling or referral to a counselor who specializes in sexual counseling for the handicapped;

— assist pt. to retain roles & tasks as much as possible within existing limitations;

— know that chronic illness has vacillations between remission & control of illness with a decrease in symptoms, & exacerbations & extension of illness with increase in symptoms;

— be prepared to support pt. emotionally & with comfort measures & treatment of acute symptoms during exacerbations; pt. may fear further disability, pain, increased dependence, & death; see NCPG #1:28, "The Patient Experiencing Fear."

3) Referral to Follow-up Care and Supervision

The patient receives referrals for follow-up care and supervision:

— begin planning for discharge on the day of admission; the pt.'s functional potential should be estimated & continually assessed so that discharge plans can be made by health care team;

— give pt. increased support when discharge is near; many pts. experience some "separation anxiety" & have concerns about leaving hospital;

— assess attitudes & concerns of family members; family therapy may be indicated for rejection & avoidance;

— send ADL assessment home or to extended care facility so that visiting nurse or staff will be able to reinforce independent progress in ADL;

— advise pt. & family of Rehabilitation Services Administration which provides diagnosis, treatment, counseling, training, & placement services to help the pt. towards vocational objectives;

— inform pt. of voluntary & self-help groups in community;

— tell pt. & family about the Directory of National Information Sources on Handicapping Conditions and Related Services (contains abstracts and addresses of 270 organizations offering services, information, and resources to handicapped individuals); obtain a copy from Superintendent of Documents, Government Printing Office, Washington, DC 20420.

Discharge Planning and Teaching Objectives/Outcomes

1) (Patient/Family/Significant Other) Can describe in own words chronic disease process and medical treatment plan, including action and side effects of medication, exercise program, diet, etc.

2) Can identify symptoms or side effects of medications which should be reported to physician right away.
3) Can describe rehabilitation program and adapt to limitations of chronic illness.
4) Knows appropriate support services and how to contact (e.g., social worker, rehabilitation services, self-help groups, etc.)

Recommended References

"The Chronic Mentally Ill in the Community—Case Management Models," by J. Lanoil. *Psychosocial Rehabilitation Journal*, Spring/Summer 1980: 1–60.

"Disability, Home Care, and the Care Taking Role in Family Life," by A.J. Davis. *Journal of Advanced Nursing*, September 1980: 475–484.

"Effects of Hospitalization: Part C: Prolonged Confinement." *NCP Guide #1:42*, 2nd Ed., Nurseco, 1980.

"Hazards of Immobility." *NCP Guide #2:45*, 2nd Ed., Nurseco, 1980.

"Mutual Withdrawal . . . the Powerful Effects of Nursing Relationships on Very Difficult and Intractable Patient Behavior," by A.T. Slavensky et al. *Perspectives in Psychiatric Care*, September/October, 1980: 194–203.

"The Patient Experiencing a Body Image Disturbance." *NCP Guide #2:29*, 2nd Ed., Nurseco, 1980.

"The Patient Experiencing Fear." *NCP Guide #1:28*, 2nd Ed., Nurseco, 1980.

"The Patient Experiencing Powerlessness." *NCP Guide #5:34*, Nurseco, 1981.

"The Patient Experiencing a Threat to Self Esteem." *NCP Guide #5:32*, Nurseco, 1981.

"The Patient Manifesting Denial." *NCP Guide #1:24*, 2nd Ed., Nurseco, 1980.

"Political Advocacy for the Chronic Mental Disabled," by C. Bellamy et al. *Psychosocial Rehabilitation Journal*, Spring/Summer 1980: 7–11.

"Problem Solving." *NCP Guide #5:47*, Nurseco, 1981.

"Psychosocial Aspects of Chronic Illness in Children," by J. Assacs et al. *Journal of School Health*, August 1980: 318-321.

"Range of Motion Exercises." *NCP Guide #1:47*, 2nd Ed., Nurseco, 1980.

"Responses to Loss: The Grief and Mourning Process." *NCP Guide #1:31*, 2nd Ed., Nurseco, 1980.

"Teaching Patients: General Suggestions." *NCP Guide #1:49*, 2nd Ed., Nurseco, 1980.

"Teaching Patients: Specific Plan for Skills and Procedures." *NCP Guide #1:50*, 2nd Ed., Nurseco, 1980.

The Patient Experiencing Guilt

Definition: Guilt is a subjective feeling of remorse and self-reproach stemming from a belief that one has done wrong, or has transgressed a social or moral code, or value system.

LONG TERM GOAL: The patient will express and explore guilt feelings and will develop alternative ways of coping with the situation that produced the guilt.

General Considerations:
— Social and moral codes develop early in life from interaction with significant others; cultural, ethnic, religious, and family values are internalized.
— The mature and well-adjusted person can discriminate between current adult situations and past childhood situations to update and affirm values.

— **Behavioral manifestations** and feelings of guilt may include:
  - feelings of remorse or regret;
  - feelings of disgrace and dishonor;
  - expectation of reproach from significant others;
  - self-punishment;
  - preoccupation with situation;
  - labels self in negative way;
  - inability to forgive self;
  - excessive stress level.

— **Causes** of guilt in a hospital setting may include:
  - patient believes that s/he has actually or potentially injured self or another person by accident or neglect;
  - patient has physically or emotionally abused someone else;
  - patient has given birth or parented child with genetic or birth defect;
  - noncompliance with health care plan.

— Repentance tasks allow the individual to repent or apologize for wrongdoing and be forgiven by significant others, social or religious group. The process of repentance facilitates self-forgiveness.
— The healthy person learns from mistakes and modifies behaviors with integrity to avoid transgressing values and moral codes.

Specific Considerations, Potential Patient Outcomes, and Nursing Actions:

1) Immediate Response to Recognition of Guilt

The patient will express feelings of guilt, remorse, and self-reproach:
— observe for excessive stress level; assist pt. to use adaptive coping mechanisms to obtain relief from stress; see NCPG #5:49, "Stress Management;"
— make frequent intermittent contact with the pt., both verbal & non-verbal to offer support, build rapport and trust relationships;
— offer self as non-judgmental listener; encourage expression of feelings; reflect & summarize pt's. words, e.g., "You seem to feel as though you could have prevented your stroke. Tell me more about that," or "You wish you hadn't spoken so sharply to your daughter?" or "Sounds like you can't forgive yourself for not going to the doctor when you first found the lump."

2) Identification of Values and Moral Codes

The patient will identify the moral code or value system transgressed:
— allow pt. to talk about transgression;
— encourage pt. to identify moral code or value system s/he has transgressed;
— identify source of moral code or value in life experience, i.e., family, culture, religion;
— explore pt.'s present value system;
— check reality of transgression: was it real or fantasy?
— support realistic assessment of the situation;
— explore ways to repent or apologize for real transgression, e.g., is pt. willing to talk about incident with daughter to validate that she perceived her mother as "talking sharply"? Is pt. sorry? Is she willing to tell daughter she is sorry and ask forgiveness? Is she willing to forgive herself? Pt. may repent by being "good pt." and by cooperating with treatment plan, physical therapy, diet, medications, etc.

3) Alternative Coping Methods

The patient will develop new ways of coping with the transgression:
— assess for lack of knowledge about defense mechanisms & responses to loss & grief; health teach as needed;
— assist pt. to identify other persons who may be available to share common problems;
— encourage pt. to discuss feelings & values with trusted person; help pt. to reach out for emotional support;
— know that self-forgiveness is an important component of mental health; emphasize the need for realistic expectations for

self & others; see NCPG #5:35, "The Patient Experiencing Shame/Embarrassment" & #5:32, "The Patient Experiencing a Threat to Self-Esteem;"
— discuss & problem solve alternative ways of behaving in situations which produced guilt; explore pros & cons of these new ways, & encourage pt. to anticipate his response to them; see NCPG #5:47, "Problem Solving;"
— observe for continued high stress level or continued unresolved feelings of guilt; refer to chaplain or psychiatric nurse specialist.

Discharge Planning and Teaching Objectives/Outcomes
1) (Patient/Family/Significant Other) Can identify situations in which s/he feels guilty.
2) Has developed alternative ways of adaptively coping with guilt feelings.

Recommended References
"The Effect of Hospitalization on Guilt and Shame Feelings." by Ilhan M. Ermutlu. *Psychiatric Forum*, Winter 1977:18–23.
"Guilt and the Working Mother." by S.L. Rad. *American Baby*, January 1980:54–55.
"The Patient Experiencing Shame Embarrassment." *NCP Guide #5:35*, Nurseco, 1981.
"The Patient Experiencing a Threat to Self-Esteem." *NCP Guide #5:32*, Nurseco, 1981.
Patient Problems in Self-Esteem and Nursing Intervention, by Merle Mishel. Los Angeles: California State University Press, 1976:52–53, 118.
"Problem Solving." *NCP Guide #5:47*, Nurseco, 1981.
"Shame." by Silvia Lange. *Behavioral Concepts & Nursing Intervention*, Carolyn Carlson & Betty Blackwell, Eds. Philadelphia: J.B. Lippincott Co., 1978:54–71.
"Spiritual Dimensions of Nursing Practice." by Jean Stallwood and Ruth Stoll. *Clinical Nursing*, Irene Beland & Joyce Passos, Eds. New York: Macmillan, 1975:1086–1089.
"Stress Management." *NCP Guide #5:49*, Nurseco, 1981.

The Patient Experiencing a Threat to Self-Esteem

Definition: **Self-esteem** is the perception or evaluation of oneself based on the quality of relationships with significant others, life experiences, and body image.

Body image is an inner sense of identity which includes body functions, abilities, and limitations.

A **threat** to self-esteem can be any event which negatively alters the individual's perception or evaluation of self.

LONG TERM GOAL: The patient will be able to cope adaptively with a threat to self-esteem and maintain/regain a realistic perception of self.

General Considerations:

— **Common causes** of a threat to self-esteem include:
  - loss of significant other due to divorce, death, or disagreement;
  - body image disturbance due to real or anticipated loss of body part or function (see NCPG #2:29, "Body Image Disturbance");
  - role change, such as change in family or work role, well role to sick role (see NCPG #5:36, "Adapting to Sick Role");
  - chronic illness with limitations and lifestyle changes; and
  - aging.

— **Common behaviors** of a threat to self-esteem include:
  - moderate to high anxiety (see NCPG #1:22, "Anxiety");
  - negative labeling of self—example, "I'm just a burden," "I'm only a housewife," "I'm stupid;"
  - devaluing of self; feels unliked, unloveable;
  - tendency to withdraw by removing self from social situations, avoiding threatening subjects or situations; may be fearful, rigid;
  - tendency to submit and be passive, non-assertive, compliant;
  - aggressive and hostile behaviors; mistrust;
  - feels powerless and unable to see alternatives in situations; and
  - use of defense mechanisms such as denial, intellectualization.

— **Nursing responsibilities** include assessing patient for behaviors associated with threat to self-esteem, choosing interventions to facilitate coping with the threat, and providing anticipatory guidance for coping with future threats.

Specific Considerations, Potential Patient Outcomes, and Nursing Actions:

1) Immediate
Response to
Recognition of
Threat to Self-
Esteem

The patient will be able to explore feelings, perception of self, and source of threat:
- provide openings for pt. to express feelings by validating your observations (e.g., "You look upset . . . what is happening with you?");
- accept pt.'s feelings & explore further; focus on pt.'s perception of self & events; do not challenge unrealistic perceptions or defensive behaviors;
- listen for & assist pt. to identify the sources of the threats; utilize reality testing to evaluate the perception of the threat (e.g., does pt. have correct information? Does pt. perceive his own abilities accurately? Is there some past experience that makes this situation threatening?); identify & explore distortion of reality;
- validate own knowledge of the components of the threatening situation with health team, pt., physician, chart, & textbooks (e.g., prognosis, treatment, side effects, etc.);
- offer safe, supportive atmosphere of respect & calm attentiveness to pt. needs & concerns; provide for basic needs and activities of daily living (ADL);
- assess anxiety level & facilitate coping with anxiety (see NCPG #1:22);
- assess for knowledge of appropriate behaviors of current health role & health teach as needed (see NCPGs #5:36. "Sick Role" & #5:30, "Chronic Illness Role").

2) Restoration to
Adaptive
Coping

The patient will explore own strengths and past coping mechanisms; the patient will plan ADL:
- explore past coping mechanisms & abilities; assist pt. to generalize from past, successful coping to present threat situation; focus on strengths & assets;
- allow pt. to make as many decisions as possible in ADL (e.g., planning time of treatments, ambulation, hold visitors phone, selecting menu);
- give positive reinforcement, using words & active listening, as pt. explores strengths & makes decisions on ADL;
- involve significant others & family to support pt. in adaptive coping with threat by non-judgmental listening, acceptance, hopeful attitude, & touch;
- assess pt.'s knowledge of relaxation techniques & health teach as needed; encourage diversionary activities, hobbies, exercise as appropriate to pt.'s physical condition.

3) Anticipatory Guidance to Future Threats	The patient will problem solve for alternative options to cope with threat to self-esteem:

    — problem solve to explore pros & cons of alternative coping responses (refer to NCPG #5:47, "Problem Solving"); role play to practice alternative behaviors in small units so that the pt. can select most adaptive coping response & experience success;

    — explore pt.'s negative expectations with him, focusing on questioning: Why do I have this expectation? Where does it come from? What person in my past (mother, father, friend) would agree with this negative expectation? What purpose does it serve? Does it realistically describe my here-and-now experiences?

    — facilitate anticipation of possible future threats; using role playing & behavioral rehearsal, assist pt. to cope effectively in behavioral trial runs;

    — reinforce, using words & behavior, realistic, positive anticipation of coping effectively with threat;

    — assess learning needs for communications of feelings & ideas, for asking to have needs met; teach communication skills & assertion techniques as needed;

    — teach pt. to develop positive affirmations about self, such as "I am flexible and calm," "I am a person who can learn and grow," "I am growing stronger and healthier," "I can learn from difficult relationships and situations."

Discharge Planning and Teaching Objectives/Outcomes

1) (Patient/Family/Significant Other) Can recognize and demonstrate increased ability to cope with threat to self-esteem.
2) Can describe a realistic perception of self.

Recommended References

"Becoming An Assertive Nurse," by D. Bakdash. *American Journal of Nursing*, October 1978:1710–1712.

"Developing a Child's Self-Esteem," by R. Fleming. *Pediatric Nursing*, July–August 1979:58–60.

"The Patient Experiencing a Body Image Disturbance." *NCP Guide #2:29*, 2nd Ed., Nurseco, 1980.

"The Patient Experiencing Anxiety." *NCP Guide #1:22*, 2nd Ed., Nurseco, 1980.

"The Patient Adapting to Chronic Illness Role." *NCP Guide #5:30*, Nurseco, 1981.

"The Patient Adapting to the Sick Role." *NCP Guide #5:36*, Nurseco, 1981.

Patient Problems in Self-Esteem and Nursing Intervention by Merle Mishel. Los Angeles: California State University Press. 1976.

"Problem Solving." *NCP Guide #5:47*, Nurseco, 1981.

"Reminiscence, Self-Esteem and Self–Other Satisfactions in Adult Male Alcoholics," by D. Gibson. *Journal of Psychiatric Nursing*, March 1980:7–11.

"Self-Concept and Mastectomy," by H. Jenkins. *Journal of Geriatric Nursing*, January–February 1980:38–42.

"Supporting the Hospitalized Elderly Patient," by Ann Lore. *American Journal of Nursing*, March 1979:496–499.

The Patient Manifesting Noncompliance

Definition: Noncompliance in a health care setting means not adhering (or only partially adhering) to a prescribed therapeutic or disease-prevention regimen.

LONG TERM GOAL: The patient will comply with prescribed treatment or prevention regimen in a responsible, informed manner; the patient will be assisted to participate adequately in self-care and achieve maximum health potential.

General Considerations:
— **Behavioral manifestations** of noncompliance include:
  - disregards suggested health regimen
  - cooperates with some parts but does not adhere to rest of care plan
  - "forgets" appointments, medications, treatments
  - affect is distrustful, angry, fearful
  - anxiety
  - continuously postpones health care
— **Causes** can include:
  - lack of understanding of diagnosis and treatment plan
  - denial of illness and consequences
  - life-style of continual crisis
  - desire to remain ill and dependent for secondary gains
  - low self-esteem
  - home or job demands
  - cost of treatment
  - negative attitude toward health care providers
  - high stress level
  - severe symptoms due to prescribed treatment
— Compliance is enhanced by use of teaching programs, by a positive and accepting attitude on the part of health professionals, and by efforts to stimulate patient and family motivation.
— **Nursing responsibilities include** assessment of variables affecting patient's compliance and noncompliance behaviors in order to recognize and support positive coping mechanisms and achieve participation and cooperation in health care.

Specific Considerations, Potential Patient Outcomes, and Nursing Actions:

1) Immediate Response to Recognition of Noncompliance
   The patient will be able to discuss situation in which s/he was noncompliant; the patient will be accepted and valued as a unique individual:
   — listen attentively to pt.'s ideas & concerns; allow pt. to describe situation from his point of view; assess reality perception;
   — treat pt. in respectful way; approach in unhurried, relaxed manner; avoid negative criticism; ﹡

— encourage expression of feelings, i.e., "Tell me more about your concerns with the side effects of your blood pressure medication;"

— summarize & reflect back expressions of feelings, i.e., "So you're saying you were really upset/scared/angry when you heard the results of your blood test;"

— encourage pt. to define & discuss own needs; refrain from forcing treatments;

— assess for stress level, stage of loss, anxiety, negative attitudes towards health professionals, self-esteem (see recommended references);

— see NCPGs #1:21, "The Patient Manifesting Anger," #1:22, "The Patient Manifesting Anxiety," #1:24, "The Patient Manifesting Denial," & #1:28, "The Patient Experiencing Fear."

2) Restoration to Adaptive Coping

The patient will accept information about prescribed therapeutic plan; the patient will be an active participant in planning and implementing care plan; the patient will participate in self-care:

— ask questions to assess pt.'s knowledge of diagnosis, disease process, treatment plan, & specific treatments;

— explore with pt. the effects of his behavior of noncompliance on self & significant others (SOs);

— encourage mutual problem solving & interdependence; explain team approach with pt. as an important part of team;

— assess problem-solving skills & teach as needed; see NCPG #5:47, "Problem Solving;"

— invite pt. to ask questions; provide reliable information; see NCPG #1:49, "Teaching Patients: General Suggestions;"

— discuss & explain procedures in advance; do not surprise pt., prepare pt. for new situations by anticipating situation & utilizing role playing, problem solving, & behavior modification;

— give verbal & non-verbal positive reinforcement for adaptive coping & appropriate compliance;

— involve pt. in active participation in setting goals & planning care; involve family & SOs as pt. desires;

— invite pt. to express preferences, likes & dislikes as much as possible in the situation;

— encourage pt. to participate in activities of daily living (ADL) in his own way; praise for participation in self-care;

— be aware that cost of medication or treatment is often a problem for elderly, adolescents, & heads of household; make appropriate referral to social service as needed;

— consult with physician & other health team members to explore problems & plan pt. care;

— refrain from performing nonessential procedures;

— introduce pt. to other persons who have had similar experiences & have positive reactions.

Discharge Planning and Teaching Objectives/Outcomes

1) (Patient/Family/Significant Other) Can approach health professionals for consultation in health maintenance and health care.
2) Can ask for information about treatment plan, can express feelings and concerns about treatment plan.
3) Is able to explain reason for and intended effect of treatments.
4) States s/he will cooperate with treatment plan in a responsible, informed, active way.
5) Can describe dangerous effects of poor health practices, of noncompliance with prescribed regimen.

Recommended References

"Behavior Modification." *NCP Guide #5:37*, Nurseco, 1981.
"The Patient Experiencing Anger." *NCP Guide #1:21*, 2nd Ed., Nurseco, 1980.
"The Patient Experiencing Anxiety." *NCP Guide #1:22*, 2nd Ed., Nurseco, 1980.
"The Patient Experiencing Denial." *NCP Guide #1:24*, 2nd Ed., Nurseco, 1980.
"The Patient Experiencing A Threat to Self-Esteem." *NCP Guide #5:32*, Nurseco, 1981.
"Problem Solving." *NCP Guide #5:47*, Nurseco, 1981.
"Responses to Loss: The Grief and Mourning Process." *NCP Guide #1:31*, 2nd Ed., Nurseco, 1980.
"Stress Management." *NCP Guide #5:49*, Nurseco, 1981.
"Teaching Patients: General Suggestions." *NCP Guide #1:49*, 2nd Ed., Nurseco, 1980.

The Patient Experiencing Powerlessness

Definition: Powerlessness is a perceived lack of personal power or control over life events and experiences in a specific situation.

LONG TERM GOAL: The patient will experience an increased sense of power and control over life events and experiences.

General Considerations:
— **Personal power** comes from being capable, adequate and able to master the environment.
— **Powerlessness results from loss of control** over environment, self-functioning, or own behavior, and **lack of knowledge** regarding own illness or life experience, including the implications for here-and-now and future for self, family, or significant other. Loss of control may involve psychological and physiological variables.
— **Potential causes** of powerlessness include:
  - diagnosis of acute or chronic illness with disability and loss of control over body, mental ability, and independent role;
  - being a "patient" instead of usual "well" person;
  - hospitalization;
  - emergency admission due to accident or sudden acute symptoms;
  - admission to CCU or ICU;
  - developmental change with potential loss of function and abilities as in aging, or change in function and abilities as in adolescence and menopause;
  - interpersonal and relationship problems, e.g. divorce, separation, termination of a relationship, family problems;
  - actual or potential loss of significant other by death, illness, divorce, or separation; potential loss of own life due to disease process or accident;
  - dealing with insurance companies, social security, and other large organizations upon which one may be dependent for help;
  - low self-esteem, situational or chronic;
  - perception of authority figure as distant, unapproachable, talking in technical terms, non-available, not interested, not responsive.

— **Behavioral manifestations** of powerlessness include:

- frustration, discouragement
- anger, hostility
- withdrawal
- passivity
- depression
- loss of perspective

- fear
- sadness, crying
- denial
- asks many questions
- asks no questions
- inability to carry out activities of daily living

- confusion
- inability to learn
- inability to concentrate
- defensive coping mechanisms

— **Nursing responsibilities** include an awareness of potential causes, recognition of behaviors, and prescribing interventions to assist the patient to adapt to current life situation in a way that will enhance his sense of power and control.

Specific Considerations, Potential Patient Outcomes, and Nursing Actions:

1) Immediate Response to Recognition of Powerlessness

The patient will express feelings and concerns about situations in which s/he feels powerless:

— build a trust relationship by making frequent verbal & nonverbal contact with pt.; be consistent & dependable (see NCPGs #1:21, "Patient Manifesting Anger," #1:22, "Patient Experiencing Confusion," #1:24, "Patient Manifesting Denial," #1:28, "Patient Experiencing Fear");

— listen to pt.'s feelings & concerns;

— ask the pt. for his opinions, likes, dislikes, & wishes; utilize these in making care plan;

— ensure environmental *powerfulness* by putting call light, telephone, bedside stand, urinal, & other desired items within reach; be aware that hospital room & objects in it are pt.'s territory & respect his right to exert control over it.

2) Restoration of Control and Power

The patient will identify situation in which s/he feels powerless; the patient will problem solve, set goals, and try alternative adaptive behaviors to increase sense of control and power:

— promote active participation in simple & appropriate decision making in ADL such as diet preferences, time & type of hygiene measures, arrangement of physical surroundings;

— assist pt. to identify situations in which s/he feels powerless; let pt. describe situation as s/he sees it;

— provide situations in which the pt. can take control (e.g., "Would you prefer to have your dressing changed before or after lunch?" or "Would you like us to block the telephone until you're ready to receive calls?" or "How would you like your bedside stand arranged?");

— give pt. verbal & non-verbal positive reinforcement & acknowledgment for active participation in planning care in ADL, goal setting, & alternative behaviors which increase sense of power & control (e.g. verbally acknowledge that pt. made a list of questions to ask physician, asked the questions, & clarified information; or, "I see you can do your own colostomy care; how do you feel about that?" or "You have some good ideas on how to manage at home; would you like to discuss them with the discharge planning nurse?"); see NCPG #5:37, "Behavior Modification;"

— assess for readiness to assume more complicated decision making; influencing factors include severity & stability of disease process (pt. in crisis or with acute symptoms may only be able to participate in a few simple decisions), previous coping mechanisms, ability to problem solve, personality traits (passive or non-assertive persons may not know how to problem solve or make decisions); these data should be assessed before offering pt. more complicated choices; when pt. ready, utilize chart & family members to facilitate situations in which pt. can achieve increased power & control;

— assess pt.'s perception & knowledge of treatments, treatment program, diagnosis & symptoms; encourage him to express his views *before* giving information, explanation, or reassurance (e.g., "What has your doctor told you about your new medication? How do you feel about taking it? What do you expect to happen in x-ray tomorrow? How do you see yourself getting up to the bathroom at home? What do you think works the best for your back pain?");

— know that increased knowledge leads to increased sense of power; assess for learning needs & provide information PRN; see NCPGs #1:49, 50, "Teaching Patients;"

— assess pt.'s ability to problem solve & health teach as needed; include significant other & family as pt. desires; see NCPG #5:47, "Problem Solving;"

— assist pt. to direct & plan own care within the medical treatment plan; as much as safely possible, allow pt. to decide how the nurse & other health team members will participate;

— encourage pt. to ask questions; be able to say, "I don't know, but I'm willing to find out" or "I don't know; this is where you can find out;"

— assess communication patterns; assist pt. to identify own preferences, likes & dislikes, wants, feelings, values, & attitudes; reinforce clear, assertive communication of preferences & feelings to appropriate listeners; let pt. know that s/he has a choice of content & person with whom s/he communicates.

Discharge Planning and Teaching Objectives/Outcomes
1) (Patient/Family/Significant Other) Verbalizes situations in which s/he feels powerless.
2) Can describe own behaviors which enhance sense of power and control.
3) States s/he will use situational supports to take an active role in own health care.

Recommended References

"ANA Code for Nurses Revised for Greater Focus on Nurse and Client," by R.D. Hadley. *American Nurse*, October 15, 1976.

"Behavior Modification." *NCP Guide #5:37*, Nurseco, 1981.

Patient Problems in Self-Esteem and Nursing Interventions, by Merle Mishel. Los Angeles: California State University Press, 1976:61–64.

"The Patient Experiencing Confusion." *NCP Guide #1:23*, 2nd Ed., Nurseco, 1980.

"The Patient Experiencing Fear." *NCP Guide #1:28*, 2nd Ed., Nurseco, 1980.

"The Patient Manifesting Anger." *NCP Guide #1:21*, 2nd Ed., Nurseco, 1980.

"The Patient Manifesting Denial." *NCP Guide #1:24*, 2nd Ed., Nurseco, 1980.

"Problem Solving." *NCP Guide #5:47*, Nurseco, 1981.

"Teaching Patients: General Suggestions." *NCP Guide #1:49*, 2nd Ed., Nurseco, 1980.

"Teaching Patients: Specific Plan for Skills and Procedures." *NCP Guide #1:50*, 2nd Ed., Nurseco, 1980.

The Patient Experiencing Shame/Embarrassment

Definition: Shame is a subjective feeling of a sudden sense of painful self-consciousness and embarrassment, ranging from mild to intense humiliation.

LONG TERM GOAL: The patient will share feelings of shame and will participate in problem solving to avoid and manage these feelings.

General Considerations:

— Shame may be evoked by situations in which the patient experiences actual or potential loss of control or function and by invasion of body boundaries or territory; incontinence of urine or bowel movement is threatening. Shame may be experienced during admission procedures, when dressing or undressing, bathing, during examinations or treatments, while sharing a room with a stranger, or when experiencing intense feelings or pain.

— Shame can be perceived as an important self-message of conflict of values and behavior; it can provide an opportunity to: 1) increase self-awareness of attitudes and feelings, and 2) to learn alternative coping methods.

— **Characteristic behaviors** include:
  - blushing or blanching of face, neck and chest
  - avoiding eye contact, lowering eyes, blinking
  - turning face away/covering face with hands
  - hand to mouth movement
  - change in voice and speech pattern
  - twisting fingers or hands
  - nervous adjustment of hair or clothes
  - shuffling feet
  - embarrassed laugh
  - tremor in hands
  - exaggerated "chin up" (anti-shame posture)
  - patient describes feelings of embarrassment or shame
  - patient uses negative labeling of self, i.e., "I'm such a baby," "I'm dirty," "I'm dumb," "I'm disgusting."

— **Nursing responsibilities** include anticipating and preventing situations which could evoke shame or embarrassment, recognizing shame/embarrassment behaviors, intervening immediately to alleviate distress, and teaching alternative coping methods.

Specific Considerations, Potential Patient Outcomes, and Nursing Actions:

1) Prevention of Shame/Embarrassment   The patient will maintain self-respect and dignity:
   - maintain respectful & courteous relationship with pt. & family; call pt. by name, knock on door, provide privacy;
   - encourage individuality & respect differences; assess individual preferences & note on care plan;
   - explain all procedures & hospital routines; provide as much information as you think pt. wants & needs;
   - encourage pt. to anticipate new situations & explore concerns & questions;

— role-play potential situations & develop new responses;
— spend time with pt. listening to concerns, assisting pt. with ADL, & building a trust relationship;
— know that most feelings of shame can be prevented.

2) Immediate Response to Recognition of Shame

The patient will acknowledge shame/embarrassment and maintain self-respect:
— assess for non-verbal & verbal shame behaviors;
— assess pt.'s perception of self & situation;
— encourage pt. to acknowledge feelings to one other person;
— accept pt.'s feelings & validate him as a unique person;
— explore shame situation: in what way does the pt. feel embarrassed? humiliated?
— determine if hospital procedures or staff behaviors caused pt. to experience shame; if so, make amends & manage environment to prevent causes.

3) Alternative Coping Methods

The patient will develop new ways of coping with situations which evoke shame or embarrassment:
— assess pt.'s attitudes towards self & expectations of self in situation;
— teach pt. that shame/embarrassment is common & normal & often can be anticipated & prevented;
— explore "shoulds," i.e., what the pt. thinks s/he should do; support realistic expectations & correct unrealistic ones (e.g., pt. may not know expected behaviors for sick role & may feel shame at being dependent on others, sharing a bedroom with other people, exposing body for examinations, or experiencing intense feelings of fear or loss, grief & mourning);
— assess for lack of experience or skills in communication, assertiveness, or interpersonal relationships; pt. may not know how to ask for privacy or how to negotiate for special needs or wants; health teach using problem solving, behavior modification, & practice of desired behaviors (see NCPG #5:47, "Problem Solving," #5:38, "Behavior Modification," and #1:49, "Teaching Patient.");
— problem solve with pt. to restore self-respect & to avoid or change situation which evoked the shame.

Recommended References
"Behavior Modification." *NCP Guide #5:37*, Nurseco, 1981.
"The Effect of Hospitalization on Guilt and Shame Feelings," by Ilhan M. Ermutlu. *Psychiatric Forum*, Winter 1977:18–23.
"Problem Solving." *NCP Guide #5:47*, Nurseco, 1981.
"Shame," by Silvia Lange. *Behavioral Concepts and Nursing Interventions*, C. Carlson & B. Blackwell, Eds. Philadelphia: J.B. Lippincott Co., 1978:51–71.
"Stress Management." *NCP Guide #5:49*, Nurseco, 1981.
"Teaching Patients: General Suggestions." *NCP Guide #1:49*, 2nd Ed., Nurseco, 1980.

The Patient Adapting to the Sick Role

Definition: The sick role consists of the behaviors that are defined by society as appropriate to the patient's stage of illness and position on the health-illness continuum.

LONG TERM GOAL: The patient will adapt to the sick role by taking on behaviors appropriate to the current stage of illness and convalescence.

General Considerations:
— **Socialization** is a dynamic, lifelong process in which the individual acquires attitudes and values, assumes new and different roles, and learns the behaviors and skills that go with the roles.
— **Role learning and role change** take place mainly in daily interpersonal relationships. Individuals usually have several roles simultaneously including family, work, and social roles.
— There are three stages of role change in the cycle of health and illness: transition from health to illness, the period of actual illness, and convalescence.
— **Nursing responsibilities** include assessing the patient for behavioral manifestations of adaptive or maladaptive sick role, and prescribing interventions to facilitate adaptive sick role and convalescence or treat maladaptive sick role.
— **Characteristic behaviors:**

ADAPTIVE SICK ROLE	MALADAPTIVE SICK ROLE
Stage I, Transition from Health to Illness	
Recognizes symptoms; may have some shock and disbelief.	Does not recognize symptoms or completely denies symptoms.
Seeks care of health care worker or doctor.	Does not seek care of health care provider or doctor.
Tells of symptoms, problems, concerns.	Makes no mention of symptoms, problems, concerns, or exaggerates or confuses them; quiet or hyperactive.
Stage II, Actual Illness	
Participates with health care worker to plan treatment, set priorities.	Refuses to participate in treatment plan.
Complies with treatment plan.	Does not comply with treatment plan; unresponsive or negative.

Seeks relief from usual roles and responsibilities.
Asks for aid from spouse, friends, family.
Asks for acceptance of illness and love in spite of illness.

Talks about body functions and progress; preoccupied with
  self and somatic concerns.
Shares feelings and concerns; ambivalent with dependency,
  both grateful and resentful.
Asks for help appropriately from staff.

Stage III, Convalescence
  Asks for guidance in resuming previous roles and responsibilities.

Asks for help from spouse, friends, family, and co-workers in
  resuming previous tasks.
Anticipates needs and asks for convalescent medication,
  treatment, activity, and rest orders.
Convalesces and returns to previous state of health.

Continues with usual roles and responsibilities inappropriately.
Does not request aid; does everything or nothing.
Defensive or aggressive, passive-aggressive behaviors; may
  be seductive toward staff.
Complains constantly and does not acknowledge progress;
  negative or denies concerns or problems.
Does not express or seem aware of own feelings.

Asks for care from others which s/he is capable of doing for
  self, or will not ask for help; demands, withdraws,
  complains constantly.

Does not ask for guidance; assumes roles and responsibilities
  prematurely or not at all.
Does not ask for help; does too much, too little for self; resents
  offers of help.
Does not think ahead and refuses to discuss treatment plan for
  convalescence.
Refuses to give up sick role; perceives self as sick when care
  givers perceive as convalescent or healthy.

Specific Considerations, Potential Patient Outcomes, and Nursing Actions:

1) Stage I,
Transition from
Health to
Illness

The patient moves adaptively from health to illness by recognizing and reporting symptoms and by seeking care of health
worker:
— establish self as a concerned & helpful professional who wants to understand pt. & family & their concerns; encourage the
    pt. to describe symptoms & share feelings, concerns;
— orient the pt. & family to immediate environment; answer questions;

— assess pt.'s knowledge of procedures & health teach as needed, giving descriptions with simple, non-tension producing words; include what the pt. will feel, hear, see, taste, experience;

— assess pt. & family for behaviors of anxiety & fear; these may include excessive demands, refusal to cooperate, withdrawal, not asking questions; see NCPGs #1:22, "The Patient Experiencing Anxiety" & #1:28, "The Patient Experiencing Fear;"

— assess pt. for behaviors of shock & disbelief, denial, & other behaviors of loss; listen & give emotional support, accepting the pt.'s need to cope with the situation at his own pace; see NCPGs #1:24, "The Patient Manifesting Denial" & #1:31, "Responses to Loss: The Grief and Mourning Process."

2) Stage II, Actual Illness

The patient adapts to sick role by participating in setting goals and planning care; the patient cooperates with the treatment plan:

— assess pt. & family goals, priorities, & preferences; include these in care plan; work with pt. to set goals & plan care; offer support & information as needed;

— discuss concerns pt. may have with letting go of usual family, work, or social roles & responsibilities; encourage pt. to ask for help from spouse, family, & friends;

— encourage pt. to ventilate feelings & concerns about illness, hospitalization, body functions, progress, prognosis; accept feelings & preoccupation with somatic concerns;

— assess pt.'s knowledge of diet, medications, treatments, activity, rest, & diagnosis; health teach as needed;

— encourage pt. to do appropriate self-care; offer emotional support & praise; see NCPG #5:37, "Behavior Modification;"

— be aware that pt. may have lost independence & self-esteem as a result of illness & hospitalization; accept ambivalent feelings of gratitude & resentment towards staff, family, friends.

3) Stage III. Convalescence

The patient makes transition from illness to convalescence by participation in and cooperation with convalescent treatment plan:

— discuss progress & anticipate convalescence with pt. & family;

— assist pt. to resume roles & responsibilities as appropriate; encourage pt. to ask for help from staff, spouse, friends, family, co-workers;

— using anticipatory guidance, assist pt. to plan for discharge from hospital; problem solve & health teach as needed to be sure pt. & family understand discharge orders such as medication, treatments, activity, rest, diet, when to call physician; see NCPG #5:47, "Problem Solving;"

— assist pt. & family to explore community resources such as VNA, "Meals on Wheels," hospital equipment rental, homemaker service, Cancer Society, Colostomy Club (or other self-help groups);

— ask open-ended questions such as, "How do you plan to manage . . . ? "What are your plans for . . . ?"

Discharge Planning and Teaching Objectives/Outcomes

1) (Patient Family Significant Other) Can recognize appropriate behaviors in illness and convalescence.

2) Can describe plan for adapting to possible future sick role.

Recommended References

"Behavior Modification." *NCP Guide #5:37.* Nurseco. 1981.

"The Effects of Hospitalization: Part A. Tension Producing Causes." *NCP Guide #1:40.* 2nd Ed., Nurseco. 1980.

"The Effects of Hospitalization: Part B: Assessment." *NCP Guide #1:41.* 2nd Ed., Nurseco. 1980.

"The Effects of Hospitalization: Part C: Prolonged Confinement." *NCP Guide #1:42.* 2nd Ed., Nurseco. 1980.

"The Patient Experiencing Anxiety." *NCP Guide #1:22.* 2nd Ed., Nurseco. 1980.

"The Patient Experiencing Fear." *NCP Guide #1:28.* 2nd Ed., Nurseco. 1980.

"The Patient Manifesting Denial." *NCP Guide #1:24.* 2nd Ed., Nurseco. 1980.

"Problem Solving." *NCP Guide #5:47.* Nurseco. 1981.

"Responses to Loss: The Grief and Mourning Process." *NCP Guide #1:31.* 2nd Ed., Nurseco. 1980.

"Symptom Reports and Illness Behavior Among Employed Women and Homemakers." by N.F. Woods et al. *Journal of Community Health.* Fall 1979:36–45.

Behavior Modification

Definitions:
— **Behavior modification** is a teaching technique for dealing with behavioral problems; the purpose is to assist individuals to modify behavior that stands in the way of health and well-being.
— **Target behaviors** are those observable and measurable behaviors that have been identified as behavior problems.
— **Terminal behaviors** are the desired new behaviors to be learned.
— **Contingency** is a term that refers to the relationship between a behavior and the events that follow the behavior.
— **Positive reinforcement** means a desired response or behavior is followed by a positive or desired consequence; reinforcement works best when applied immediately.
— **Aversive consequences** are undesirable consequences and can be used to decrease occurrence of behavior.
— **Shaping** is the breaking down of desired terminal behaviors into a sequence of steps and rewarding each successive approximation of the steps.
— **Generalization** is the transfer of an already learned response to another situation.
— **Behavioral objectives** describe in a measurable way the behavior that the learner tries to learn; they permit an ongoing evaluation of the treatment goals (see NCPG #1:48, "Steps in Writing a Nursing Care Plan," Step 3). Example: The patient will swim or walk briskly 15 minutes every day.

General Considerations:
— **Behavioral theory** indicates that both positive and negative behaviors are learned and that behavior can be modified. Behavior modification includes principles of teaching and learning. The basic tenet of behavioral theory is: *behavior that is reinforced tends to be repeated.* Reinforcement should be given *each time* the behavior occurs; *after* the behavior is established, intermittent reinforcement (e.g. every 2–3 times) maintains the behavior *better* than reinforcement every time.
— The patient should be involved in setting goals and objectives and agree to cooperate with the plan; if the patient has limited capacity to understand this procedure, discuss the information with him in simple terms which he can understand.
— Involving the patient encourages participation, self-motivation, self-care, and limits threats to personal freedom and infringement on human rights. (See NCPG #1:49, "Teaching Patients.")
— **Nursing responsibilities** include assessing the patient for behavioral problems that interfere with health and well-being, and contracting with patient to set goals and objectives for behavior modification.

— **Behavior modification consists of six steps:**

Step 1 Define the behavior to be modified.

1.1 Identify problem behavior which needs intervention; behavior should be observable and measurable. This behavior is called the *target* behavior.

1.2 Determine how this behavior interferes with care, health, and the patient's well-being. Example: Patient is 50 pounds overweight, has erratic diet habits, and wants to lose weight as part of treatment plan to decrease blood pressure.

Step 2 Measure the behavior to be modified.

2.1 Gather baseline data, i.e., how many times does the behavior occur in a specific time period? Example: Instruct patient to keep diet diary and write down everything s/he eats for one week.

2.2 Observe sequence and pattern of behavior; example: Patient's weight is 190 lbs; daily diet diary indicates no breakfast, a high calorie 10 AM snack, a sandwich and malt for lunch, peanuts and wine at 5 PM, and a large dinner with dessert at 8 PM.

Step 3 Analyse current contingencies that maintain problem behavior or lack of ability, knowledge, or experience.

3.1 Assess for events that precede and follow behavior; pay attention to feelings as well as to who, what, when, how, and why.

3.2 Involve the patient and family in this analysis; encourage the patient to count and keep track of behavior and feelings that accompany it by keeping a journal, diary, or chart.

3.3 Assess for deficits in behavioral repertoire; these may be skills and abilities which the patient has not learned or is not currently using. Example: Patient eats to give self treat; does not know how to nurture self in other ways. Gets up too late for breakfast and eats lunch out because there is nothing in the house to take for lunch. Eats dinner late to eat with husband. Snacks to cope with anxiety and depression. Willing to work on anxiety and depression by learning new ways to cope.

Step 4 Construct program to change behavior in desired directions.

4.1 Set and write out behavioral objectives to modify the target behavior to the desired terminal behavior; include the setting or conditions under which the desired behavior is expected to occur, the specific desired behavior that can be observed and measured, and the criterion for how and when the behavior will be performed.

4.2 Include the patient in setting goals and planning program; the patient can help select appropriate positive reinforcers and suitable aversive consequences.

4.3 Nursing behaviors for positive reinforcement should include spending time with patient, verbal praise and encouragement, smiling, showing interest in discussion of specific subjects, providing opportunity for patient to have special experiences or treats.

4.4 Aversive consequences could include discontinuing special experiences or treats, participation in chores that are disliked by patient, or nursing behaviors of disinterest, frowning, turning face away, or spending less time with patient.

4.5 Teach patient that all behavior has consequences and that each individual can choose among many alternative actions and resulting consequences.

4.6 Set a specific time for trial run of program and agree to evaluate effectiveness at that time. Example: Patient will reduce diet intake to ingest 1200 calories a day, which will include 3 meals plus two snacks and a well-balanced diet. Patient will weigh in once a week and will be able to plan and have a non-food treat (flowers, music, new clothes, perfume) each time s/he loses 5 pounds. Patient will swim or walk 15 minutes daily. If no weight lost or if weight gained, patient agrees to clean out garage or wash down walls for neighbor.

Step 5 Use therapeutic instructions (expectancy).

5.1 Offer specific plan to practice modified behavior; encourage attitude of positive and matter-of-fact expectance that modified behavior will occur. Example: Plan acceptable diet and snacks with some unusual low-calorie treats; plan shopping to include items for breakfast and lunch.

5.2 Break behavior into small steps in a sequence pattern; plan practice of small steps.

5.3 Include some known desired behaviors that cannot be done simultaneously with target behavior. Example: Play guitar or flute instead of snacking; chew gum while cooking dinner instead of tasting food; folk dance or swim instead of drinking alcohol.

Step 6 Practice desired behavior, step by step.

6.1 Begin with known steps and then attempt unknown or new steps; choose simple, unthreatening situations and then gradually include more complex and difficult ones.

6.2 Instruct patient to keep diary or journal of practice, including log of new steps and modified behavior, plus feelings and concerns. Steps might include: Buy low-calorie acceptable food, prepare lunch the night before, get up early to eat breakfast, take guitar/flute lessons, prepare and eat low-calorie, well-balanced meals, keep a journal of all food ingested plus feelings and concerns.

Step 7 Reinforce small, discrete steps in adaptive direction (shaping).

7.1 Provide information of behavior change to patient, verbally and with charts.

7.2 Reinforce progress, using plan of positive reinforcement; ensure that each step taken toward the terminal/expected behavior is reinforced.

7.3 Involve family and friends in giving feedback and encouragement for steps in adaptive direction. Appreciation is not only much appreciated at this point, but also helps shape the desired behavior.

7.4 Involve patient in keeping own record or chart of desired terminal behavior, thus increasing awareness of own behavior and allowing for increased intrinsic motivation. Example: Patient can keep own weight chart and could negotiate with husband, friend, or co-worker to give verbal encouragement. Nurse can give praise and encouragement plus listen attentively to concerns, read patient's journal, and discuss patterns.

Step 8 Generalize terminal behavior to natural environment using natural reinforcers.

8.1 Assist patient to transfer modified behavior to other similar situations and environments by role playing and using problem-solving method.

8.2 Explore and anticipate with patient the natural positive reinforcement that could be expected or planned for with modified behavior. Example: Anticipate and role play dining out situations in which patient asks for fresh fruit or vegetable substitute for high-calorie item. Anticipate camping trip or vacationing with 1200 calorie diet. Encourage patient to imagine self buying smaller sized vacation clothes and having more energy and lower blood pressure.

Recommended References

"Anorexia Nervosa: Patient Behavioral Approach," By S.B. Steckel. *American Journal of Nursing,* August 1980:1471–1472.

"Behavior Modification with a Mentally Retarded Child," by M.J. Roberts et al. *American Journal of Nursing,* April 1980: 679–680.

"Contracting with Patient—Selected Reinforcers," by S.B. Steckel. *American Journal of Nursing,* September 1980:1596–1599.

"Peer Analysis of Interpersonal Responsiveness and Plan Encouraging Reshaping—Pair/Peer," by M.E. Davidson et al. *Journal of Nursing Education,* February 1980:8–12.

"Promoting Urine Control in Older Adults," by D. Mandelstam et al. *Geriatric Nursing,* November/December 1980:251–257.

"Therapeutic Tasks—Strategies for Change," by C. Goldberg. *Perspectives in Psychiatric Care,* July/August 1980: 156–162.

"Toward Reducing Stress in the Institutionalized Elderly—Therapeutic Tape Recordings," by M.M. Alvermann. *Journal of Gerontological Nursing,* November/December 1979:21–26.

"A Weight Reduction Model for Mildly Retarded Adults Living in Semi-Independent Care Facilities," by A.F. Rotalovi et al. *Journal of Advanced Nursing,* March 1980:179–186.

Birth Control: Permanent Methods

Definition: Sterilization is an operation to remove the possibility of pregnancy or to render the person incapable of conception.

GOAL: The person will be able to virtually eliminate risk of pregnancy.

General Considerations:
- **Incidence:** voluntary sterilizations in the US exceed 1.1 million per year; about two-thirds are hysterectomies and nearly one-third are vasectomies; tubal ligation type operations are growing in popularity. Abortions, while not preventing pregnancy, are used as a major means of birth control by a growing number of women; there are over 1.6 million abortions per year in the US alone.
- **Advantages:** relief from worry and inconvenience of other birth control methods; relief from unwanted pregnancy and childbirth; a cessation of transmission of hereditary diseases.
- **Disadvantages:** nearly always permanent and irreversible consequences; with microsurgical and experienced surgical techniques, it is now possible sometimes to reconnect fallopian tubes or vas deferens in men, but surgery is difficult, expensive and successful in only a small percentage of cases.
- **Counseling** should be done with both sexual partners. There should be a complete exploration of feelings re: sexuality and sterility, possibilities of divorce and re-marriage, loss of child-bearing potential and psychological consequences, especially if there is a loss of an offspring, and any pressures or influences affecting decision. Postponement or cancellation of operation is advisable if there are any signs of emotional, economic or marital stress that signal doubt, distrust or absence of free, informed consent. After open and honest discussion, there should be complete understanding and acceptance of operation, its meaning and its effect on both partners.
- **Legal Consent:** Person must be over 21, fully aware and free of influences of drugs or coercion. While sterilization is now legal in all fifty states, policies and practices vary with local governments, doctors, hospitals, and insurance or Social Service Dept. guidelines. Written consent of marital partner is usually necessary.
- Literature is available from Association for Voluntary Sterilization, Inc., 708 Third Avenue, New York, NY 10017 and from local chapters of Planned Parenthood Federation of America. Teaching aids, counseling services, diagnostic tests for pregnancy and/or venereal disease, and physician referrals are also available from the latter as well as from local free clinic, Public Health Dept. or county clinic and student health clinic.

Methods:

1) **Hysterectomy**
   - Hysterectomy is removal of uterus: total (including tubes and ovaries) or sub-total (only the uterus), also known as a partial hysterectomy.
   - Refer to NCPG #1:12, "The Patient with a Hysterectomy."

2) **Laparoscopy and Cauterization or Clips for Tubes**
   - The insertion of a laparoscope through a small, one inch incision near the navel for purpose of viewing fallopian tubes that are then commonly cauterized (some doctors use clips).
   - Carbon dioxide gas is pumped into abdomen to facilitate lifting and viewing tubes. Frequently this remains in abdomen to be gradually absorbed. "Post insufflation syndrome" is the name for any resulting severe pain in chest, shoulder, and neck that patient experiences. Analgesic injections are often required to reduce discomfort and the normal 12 hour hospitalization may be prolonged. Some surgeons are now using a laparoscope "key" device to remove CO_2 before closing incision and this has been helpful.
   - Effectiveness: About 1 in 1,000 women can get pregnant after this type surgery. Cauterization makes this operation nearly always permanent, so clips are occasionally used for younger women.
   - Complications include: hemorrhage, infection, cardiopulmonary problems in about 1-5 per 100 cases.
   - Nursing care is similar to that of a patient with a mini-lap tubal ligation (see NCPG #5:19) although the surgery and hospitalization are often shorter. Most women recover in a few days from the sore throat (from general anesthetic tube), sore stomach, and mild to moderate cramps. Menstrual periods, hormone levels, and sexual abilities are unchanged.

3) **Tubal Ligation/Mini-Laparotomy**
   - A tubal ligation via mini-laparotomy is a small incision between the navel and the pubis for the purpose of cutting the fallopian tubes in half and tying them off.
   - Refer to NCPG #5:19, "The Patient with a Tubal Ligation (via Mini-Laparotomy)."

4) **Vasectomy**
   - Vasectomy is the resection bilaterally of the vas deferens or ducts that carry sperm from the testes to the penis.
   - Effectiveness: More than 99.5%; however, complete sterility may not be attained until several weeks or months after surgery. Other methods of birth control are necessary until follow-up sperm counts are negative. Operation is usually not reversible, and even if the tubes are re-connected, restored fertility is only 20% likely because sperm antibodies (which develop in many

men) lessen chances.
- Advantages: quick (10-20 minute operation under local anesthetic in an office or clinic), requires no hospitalization (only a couple of days rest with ice packs and elevation of scrotum), does not affect hormones, erections, climaxes, or ejaculations (except rarely — perhaps 5 per 1,000 men), sexual pleasure is same or increased.
- Complications are usually minor, self-limiting and arise in less than 10% of cases. These include: bleeding, hematoma inflammation, infection, ecchymosis (bruise), persistent swelling (due to epididymitis or spermatic granuloma). Aspirin, scrotal supports, ice or heat packs and occasionally, antibiotics, will be used PRN.

5) **Abortion**
- Abortion is the termination of pregnancy before the fetus is theoretically viable.
- Kinds: spontaneous, also called miscarriage, happens when natural body processes end pregnancy before birth — usually before the 20th week of pregnancy; induced abortion is a medical procedure used to end pregnancy.
- Legality: now legal in every state since the Supreme Court decision of 1973; abortions after the first trimester are subject to local state regulation and hospital policies.
- Induced abortion is currently used by many women as a substitute for other methods of contraception. Although a relatively safe procedure performed by a skilled doctor in the first trimester, it is not without some risk of hemorrhage, infection, and serious pyschological consequences. After the first trimester, abortions are much more dangerous, difficult, and expensive. Repeated abortions may increase the possibility of premature births in later, desired pregnancies.
- Refer to NCPGs #3:01, "The Patient Having an Abortion" and #3:02, "The Patient with a D & C (Dilatation and Curretage)."

Recommended References
All About Vasectomy (Rev. August, 1978). Planned Parenthood Federation of America, Inc., 810 Seventh Avenue, New York, NY 10019.
"The Patient Having an Abortion." *NCP Guide #3:01,* Nurseco, 1978.
"The Patient with a D & C (Dilatation and Curretage)." *NCP Guide #3:02,* Nurseco, 1978.
"The Patient with a Hysterectomy." *NCP Guide #1:12,* 2nd Ed., Nurseco, 1980.
"The Patient with a Tubal Ligation (via Mini-Laparotomy)." *NCP Guide #5:19,* Nurseco, 1981.

Birth Control: Temporary Methods

GOAL: The person(s) will be able to significantly reduce risk of pregnancy without harmful effects to self or partner.

General Considerations:
- Abstinence or continence is the only completely risk-free temporary method of birth control. Persons may choose either of these methods for various reasons: moral, religious, personal, physical, or psychosocial. In any case, the choice should be acceptable to both sexual partners and be respected by other persons, especially family and friends.
- Literature on the various methods of birth control and their relative effectiveness is available from local chapters of Planned Parenthood Federation of America. Teaching aids, counseling services, birth control aids and prescriptions, diagnostic tests for pregnancy and/or venereal disease, and physician referrals are also available from them as well as from the local "Free" clinic, the public health or county clinic, Right to Life Organizations, and student health clinics. *Hope Is Not A Method* is a recommended film (see references) which can be purchased or rented.
- Those who participate in counseling or providing birth control information and help are usually also responsible for detection of cancer, venereal disease, and for non-VD infection control activities (information, screening tests, referral for treatment, and required reports).
- Effectiveness rates are computed by subtracting failure rate from 100%; failure rates quoted are a combination of method and user failures per 100 women per year.
- **LESS RELIABLE** methods (than those listed later) include:
  - *Lactation:* breast feeding suppresses ovulation for some time, *for some women,* but the risk of pregnancy may be as high as 40%.
  - *Non-intercourse sex:* involves mutual masterbation, oral or anal copulation, interfemoral intercourse (between legs), "petting" to sexual climax (release of sperm), and/or astrological birth control. The latter involves avoiding sex each month during the sun/moon phase, corresponding to the time of one's birth. Astrologers believe, *without scientific basis,* that female eggs are released at this time.
  - *Intercourse mid-menstrual cycle:* although unlikely, it *is* possible for an egg to be in the fallopian tube at this time.
  - *Withdrawal:* involves removal of penis from vagina before ejaculation or leaking of any sperm occurs. Risk occurs if sperm is

left on the woman's thighs or pubis, as they can still swim into vagina.
- *Douching immediately after intercourse:* regardless of beliefs to the contrary, or the type of solution used (tea, vinegar, soapy water, cola, gingerale, etc.), this method is ineffective because of speed of sperm swimming into uterus before any douching can take place.
- *Plastic food wrap used like a condom:* commonly breaks, slips off, or leaks.

Bona Fide Methods, Effectiveness, Advantages, and Disadvantages:

1) **Condoms** ("rubbers," "prophylactics")
   - A thin rubber sheath, slipped over an erect penis just before intercourse.
   - Effectiveness: 64-97%, depending on correct usage; effectiveness enhanced when used with other methods (see below).
   - Advantages: inexpensive, easily available without prescription, free from major side effects, no medical supervision needed, and provides some protection from venereal disease.
   - Disadvantages: for some they may inhibit sensation, enjoyment, spontaneity, and erection; they have been known to split, tear or spill during usage; sometimes allergies to rubber necessitate usage of other, more expensive types, such as lambskin.

2) **Diaphragms**
   - A thin, dome-shaped, shallow rubber cup surrounding a metal spring rim placed over the cervical os, between rear and side walls of the vagina and behind the symphysis pubis bone.
   - Concern over side effects of "The Pill" has caused an increase in the popularity for the diaphragm; other indications for use include: inability to use an IUD; non-allergy to spermicidal preparations; acceptability, motivation, and compliance readiness of both sexual partners; satifactorily meeting anatomical, medical, and other psychological criteria; and woman's informed choice over other less desirable methods. Contraindications include: a displaced or abnormal organ and surrounding structures (e.g., uterine prolapse, retroversion, anteflexion, cystocele, rectocele, inadequate muscular support, etc.) and a sexual pattern of behavior that includes a variety of partners and positions and/or multiple intercourse.
   - Effectiveness: 70-95%, depending on correct fit and usage.
   - Correct size should be carefully supervised. Size and fit should be re-checked at yearly intervals and after a pregnancy or a 10 pound weight gain or loss.
   - Wearer should be taught to check diaphragm once a month for holes or thin spots by holding up to light. Ordinary care includes washing with mild soap and warm water, thorough rinsing and completely air drying, and dusting with cornstarch (no scented talcs or vaseline to weaken rubber). One usually lasts two years with proper care. Newer, disposable models are now

available as is a type of polyurethane sponge impregnated and bonded with spermicide and designed for several days wear at a time.
- The standard diaphragm should be inserted less than six hours prior to intercourse, preferably a shorter time, and a teaspoonful of spermicidal jelly placed in the cup prior to insertion. The woman should leave it in place at least six hours after last sex act; if intercourse occurs within this six-hour period, additional spermicidal jelly or foam should be inserted into the vagina before each act. A tampon can be inserted to absorb contraceptive and/or sexual fluids if the diaphragm needs to remain in place for a longer time before it can be conveniently removed (no longer than 24 hours, however).
- Advantages: no ill effects such as other methods cause; high effectiveness when used correctly and with spermacide every time.
  Disadvantages: possible increased incidence of bladder infections; occasional allergic reactions to rubber or spermicide; sometimes wearer finds insertion to be distasteful, inconvenient or inhibiting; repeated fittings are needed for those who gain weight or lose weight readily; dislodgement problems due to vaginal wall expansion during state of sexual arousal related to frequent penile insertions, sexual position (woman on top), or both.

3) **Cervical Caps**
   - A small, rubber, thimble-like device that fits directly over cervix and needs only a small amount of spermicide.
   - Popular in Europe, not yet approved by FDA, but available here in US from physicians and clinics participating in FDA-approved studies of effectiveness.
   - Advantages and disadvantages thought to be same as those for diaphragms.

4) **Intrauterine Devices** (IUDs)
   - A small plastic device, some with copper, that is inserted into the uterus and remains there indefinitely; some release a synthetic hormone and these need replacing once a year; a nylon string hangs out of the cervical os into the vagina, making it possible for woman to check periodically to be sure IUD is still there.
   - Effectiveness rate: 90-99%, lower for those IUDs having copper or progesterone hormone in them.
   - If a menstrual period is more than a week late, or if woman thinks she is pregnant, she should contact her doctor or clinic right away. She should never try to remove IUD herself.
   - Because of increased susceptibility to pelvic infection, wearer should be warned to note and report to MD immediately signs

of abdominal pain or tenderness, very heavy bleeding, fever, unusual vaginal discharge. Women who have a history of PID (pelvic inflammatory disease) or a variety of sexual partners should not use an IUD.
- Advantages: convenient, frees wearer of concerns associated with other birth control methods, no daily routine or precautionary activity needed at time of intercourse; cannot be felt by partners.
- Disadvantages: occasional displacement, expulsion, discomfort/pain, cramping, heavier than usual menstrual flow or irregular bleeding; increased risk of pelvic infection.

5) **Ovulation Method** (Fertility Awareness Method, Rhythm, Natural Method, Sympto-Thermal Method, Periodic Abstinence, Billings Method).
- Currently gaining in popularity as a natural method without harmful effects of chemical usage, this method has evolved into a combination of the "calendar method" (based on menstrual history), the "temperature method," and the "vaginal mucus method." It is presently known as the Sympto-Thermal Method. It involves the total abstinence from sexual intercourse during the ovulation period, which is determined specifically for each woman. It was first described by Drs. Billings in 1952.
- A chart or graph is made for each woman, noting the following on a *daily basis:*
    (a) cervical mucus secretions progressing from thick, sticky, and slightly yellow or cloudy to clear, slippery, and watery in nature;
    (b) signs of breast tenderness and/or "mittelschmerz" (lower abdominal tenderness on either side during mid-cycle); and
    (c) basal body temperatures to determine period when temperature rises and remains at consistently higher level for a few days. For most women, 96-98° (F.), orally is considered normal before ovulation and 97-99° typical after ovulation. Changes are fractional so a special *basal* thermometer that registers $1/10$ degrees is best to use.
- The "Safe" period for intercourse is then determined to be a few "dry" days following menstruation prior to the onset of the above signs and again for a period of about ten days prior to the next menstruation.
- Effectiveness: 75-98%, depending on regularity of woman's cycle, her correct observations of ovulation's signs, and the cooperation and discipline of both partners.
- Advantages: no cost (except for thermometer), easily taught by professional, experienced instructors to well-motivated persons, acceptable to all religious groups, medical check-ups or supervision not required as part of method, no chemical or mechanical interference with body processes, easy to reverse when conception is desired, and some report 98% reliability in preventing conception.

— Disadvantages: requires consistent, persistent, accurate record-keeping and the mutual cooperation and self-control of sexual partners; inhibiting to spontaneous sex; no protection from impetuous contact, rape or incest; leukorrhea may interfere with women's observations of mucus character or chronic, frequent infections with normal temperature graphs.

6) **Spermicides** (Cream, Jelly, Foam, or Suppositories)
   — Contain an inert base that provide a physical barrier to sperm and a chemical that immobilizes and kills sperm.
   — Effectiveness: 70-98%, depending on whether they are correctly inserted into vagina with applicator provided (except for suppository form), and are inserted one hour prior to intercourse. Foam is considered to be more effective than cream or jelly types; effectiveness of spermicides is enhanced when used in combination with other methods (condom, diaphragm, etc.) Douching, after intercourse, should not be done for at least six hours to allow full spermicidal activity and protection.
   — Advantages: easy to obtain in drugstore without prescription, easy to use without major harmful side effects. Foam type is thought to provide a degree of protection from some verereal diseases.
   — Disadvantages: messy, inconvenient, interferes with spontaneity of mood; allergies can occur which may or may not be corrected by changing brands; more important, there is recent evidence to indicate that increased incidence of serious birth defects may occur in those who are or have recently used spermicides.

7) **Oral Contraceptives ("The Pill")**
   — Refer to NCPG #5:42, "Drugs: Birth Control Pills."

Recommended References

Basics of Birth Control, Revised E., New York: Planned Parenthood Federation of America, Inc., 810 7th Avenue, 1980.

Birth Control Methods. San Juan, PR: Searle & Co., 1980.

Choices..., by Sheri Tepper, Denver, CO: RMPP Publication, 1952 Vine St., 1977.

"A College Contraceptive Clinic," by Susan W. Andrews. *The American Journal of Nursing*, April 1976:592-593.

Hope Is Not A Method (16 minute film). Northfield, IL: Perennial Education, Inc., 1825 Willow rd.

"Ovulation Method of Birth Control." by Barbara Timby. *The American Journal of Nursing*, June 1976:982-929.

"Teaching Successful Use of the Diaphragm," by Lynn Lesak Gorline. *The American Journal of Nursing*, October 1979:1732-1735.

"Warning on Spermicides," by Jean Seligmann, *Newsweek*, April 13, 1981:84.

Ways to Chart your Fertility Pattern, Revised Ed., New York: Planned Parenthood Federation of America, Inc., 1979.

What About Sterilization? Revised Ed., Booklet A. Sacramento, CA: California State Department of Health Services.

Recommended References

"Diet: Diarrhea Control." *NCP Guide #3:43*, Nurseco, 1977.

"A Double-Bind Trial of the Effect of Wheat Bran on Symptoms of the Irritable Bowel Syndrome," by S. Soltoft et al. *Lancet*, March 7, 1976:270-272.

"A Framework for Prevention: Changing Health Damaging to Health Generating Life Patterns," by M. Milio. *American Journal of Public Health*, May 1976:435-439.

Nutrition: Principles and Application in Health Promotion, by C. Suitor and M. Hunter. Philadelphia: J.B. Lippincott & Co., 1980.

"Treatment of Symptomatic Diverticular Disease with a High-Fibre Diet," by A. Brodribb. *Lancet*, March 26, 1977:664-666.

"Utilization of a Low-Lactose Milk," by S.J. Turner. *American Journal of Clinical Nutrition*, July 1976:739-744.

"Wrestling with the Irritable Colon," by R.P. Almy. *Medical Clinics of North America*, January 1978:203-210.

Diet: Weight Control

LONG TERM GOAL: The patient achieves and maintains ideal body weight range with sufficient balanced nutrients for high level wellness.

General Considerations:
— Weight gain is often a concern for adults who are more than 5% over their ideal body weight (IBW). The term "obese" refers to those who are more than 20% over IBW.
— Obesity has become a serious national health problem. Most American adults, it is estimated, consume nearly twice as much protein, fat, and cholesterol as recommended, or needed.
— For safe weight reduction, obese persons should be under the continuing care of *health professionals* who include an internist, a registered dietician or consulting nutritionist, and a behavioral psychologist. Dieters should beware of lay therapists who promise miraculous or quick results with programs or products to sell.
— Nearly all quick weight-loss regimens are *ketogenic* diets that deprive the body of carbohydrate energy, causing it to burn protein and producing a state of ketosis. Ketosis results in rapid water loss (often misinterpreted as fat loss), irritability, insomnia, fatigue and/or headache. A twenty-pound weight loss in a few weeks may not include more than a few ounces of fat and is likely to be regained upon return to former eating habits.
— Good weight-loss diets include a balanced diet from *all four* basic food groups, but in reduced portions to total *less* than the body's energy needs. A formula often suggested is a daily diet plan for 15-20 calories per kilogram of IBW.
— Eliminating *500 calories a day* of sweet or fatty snacks and alcoholic or high caloric beverages can result in a 3,500 calorie deficit, or a *one-pound loss, per week.*
— Weight-reducing clubs provide low-cost group counseling and mutual support. Nationally recognized ones are Weight Watchers, Overeaters Anonymous and TOPS (Take Off Pounds Sensibly). Success depends upon the individual's response to a particular group, type of therapy, or philosophy.
— Area hospitals and local universities offer weight-reduction and maintenance programs. These usually incorporate aspects of diet, exercise, psychological counseling with behavior modification, and educational classes on such topics as nutrition, calorie counting and control, binge eating, family support systems, personal values, role of emotions, assertiveness techniques, and food diaries.
— For sound nutritional information, consult various articles and books listed below under Recommended References.

- **Nursing responsibilities** are to:
  1) assist with assessment of individual's health and nutrition status (This includes a medical and dietary history; a determination of eating and behavior patterns as well as socioeconomic, ethnic, and religious factors; physical exam; x-ray and laboratory findings; and an assessment of psychological strengths, limitations and learning needs.);
  2) assist patient with problem identification, goal setting, and problem-solving plan;
  3) interpret dietary prescription;
  4) provide nutrition education, recipe modification, and meal plans; and
  5) make appropriate referrals to nutrition specialist, psychological counselor, group therapy program, and/or published sources of reliable nutrition and weight loss information.

General Rules:

1) Keep a food record or diary that includes: amount and type of food or drink consumed, with whom, when, location, type of activity or situation while eating, subjective feelings or mood, and level of hunger.
2) Weigh *only once a week,* on the same scale, in the same clothing, at the same time of day.
3) Confine all beverages to those with as few calories as possible. Include low-fat or non-fat milk, grapefruit and tomato juice, mineral water, and diet soft drinks. Drink coffee and tea plain without milk or sweeteners. Try to eliminate or significantly reduce alcoholic beverages. Avoid fruit juices such as grape, orange, or pineapple that are higher in natural sugar (fructose).
4) Eat nothing breaded, soaked in gravy or sauces, or fried in oil, shortening, butter or margarine. Meat, poultry, and fish should be baked or broiled. Vegetables should be eaten raw or cooked in steam without sugar, shortening, or sauces. Fruits should be eaten fresh, stewed in water, or canned in natural juices without syrup.
5) Choose fish over fowl, fowl over beef, and beef over pork for less fattening protein. Avoid all processed, packaged, or canned meats as well as bacon, sausage, hot dogs, and organ meats.
6) Have a fresh vegetable salad at least thirty minutes before dinner. Choose lesser calorie dressings such as lemon juice or vinegar, low-fat sour cream, or low-fat yogurt; use sparingly. Always order dressings "on the side" when dining out.
7) Use a smaller plate than usual at mealtimes. Take half portions, eat slowly, chew well (at least 10-15 times each bite), and pause 10-15 seconds between bites to assuage appetite and to finish when others at table do.
8) Choose fresh fruits for dessert or eat half portions of carefully selected, calorie-reduced, specially-prepared desserts. If a treat is very important, make allowances for it in diet plan, either fasting or cutting back temporarily to compensate.

9) Eat every three hours during day to avoid uncontrollable hunger, eating binges, and oversized meals. Snack on fresh vegetables and fruit, unbuttered popcorn, and low-calorie liquids.
10) Drink at least eight full glasses of water or liquids daily.
11) When not eating, keep food out of sight and not easily accessible. Do marketing only after a meal, never before; shop only from a list. Refrain from purchasing high-caloric snacks, non-nutritive foods, commercial mixes, and packaged foods with "hidden sugar". Read labels.
12) Train self to "make-up" for a day's "break in diet" by a day of fast. An occasional day or weekend off diet is OK, as long as it doesn't result in guilt, giving up, and subsequent overeating.
13) Exercise, it has been found, tends to *decrease* appetite in obese people. So whenever possible, (daily or several times weekly) take a walk, bike ride or swim for 20-30 minutes before a meal or instead of a usual snack time.
14) Do not become discouraged when plateaus are reached and no further weight loss is apparent. Continue on diet, increase exercise slightly and persist toward weight goal.
15) When following your ideal body weight maintenance diet, do not exercise less as you begin to eat more. With a four-pound weight gain over IBW, return to former weight reduction diet.

Discharge Planning and Teaching Objectives/Outcomes

1) (Patient/Family/Significant Other) Can explain in own terms the relationship between obesity and chronic health problems.
2) Can identify which risk factors s/he has and can tell how s/he can modify them in own favor.
3) Can state own energy and nutrient requirements.
4) Can identify own causes of weight problems (e.g., rate, frequency, and amount of eating; content of diet; emotional reasons) and tell how s/he will try to handle these.
5) Has developed own goals and personal intervention program that include desirable life-style modifications of diet, exercise, and eating patterns.
6) Has developed daily and weekly diet plans; has a contingency plan for a break in diet; has a plan to control eating in restaurants and other people's homes; and is able to accept alternative activities for uncontrolled eating.

Recommended References

"A Sensible Approach to the Obese Patient," by L. Kathleen Mahan. *Nursing Clinics of North America,* June 1979:229-245.

 Behavior Modification." *NCP Guide #5:37,* Nurseco, 1981.

Calories and Carbohydrates, 4th Rev. Ed., by Barbara Kraus. New York: The New American Library, Inc., 1981.

"Diet: Fat-Controlled, Low Cholesterol." *NCP Guide #4:43,* Nurseco, 1978.

Food Values of Portions Commonly Used, 13th Ed., by Jean Pennington and Helen Church. Philadelphia: J.B. Lippincott Co., 1981.

"General Dietary Principles for the Diabetic." *NCP Guide #1:36,* Nurseco, 1980.

Jane Brody's Nutrition Book, by Jane Brody. New York: W.A. Norton & Co., 1981.

"Nutritive Value of American Foods" (Handbook No. 456). Washington, DC: Agricultural Research Service, US Dept. of Agriculture, USDA Government Printing Office, 1975.

The Barbara Kraus 1981 Rev. Ed. Calorie Guide to Brand Names & Basic Foods by Barbara Kraus. New York: The New American Library, Inc., 1981.

"The Healthiest Way You'll Ever Lose 10 Pounds in 2 Weeks," by Edwin Bayrd. *Family Health,* July/August, 1979:28-30.

The Pritikin Permanent Weight-Loss Manual by Nathan Pritikin. New York: Grosset & Dunlap, 1981.

Think Yourself Thin by Dr. Frank J. Bruno. New York: Harper & Row, 1972.

Drugs: Birth Control Pills

GOAL: The woman will be able to minimize risk of pregnancy without seriously harmful side effects or complications.

General Considerations:

— "The Pill," as it is commonly called, usually contains two female synthetic hormones (estrogen and progestogen) that keep an egg from being released by the ovary. The estrogen suppresses secretion of Follicle Stimulating Hormones and Releasing Factors while the progestogen suppresses Luteinizing Hormones and Releasing Factors, thereby causing the cervical mucus to become more resistant to penetration and movement of sperm.

— Combination types are taken once a day for 21 days and then stopped for seven days, during which time menstrual flow occurs. The 21-day pill cycle is then repeated. Sometimes the doctor prescribes a different-colored, inert (inactive) pill to be taken during the 7-day period so that the daily pill taking habit is reinforced.

— The "Mini-Pill" is a progestogen only preparation that is taken daily on a continuous basis.

— **Effectiveness:** 99% when taken correctly *and consistently* according to directions.

— **Advantages:** most effective, temporary method of birth control; convenient, doesn't interfere with spontaneity or love-making activity; short-term (less than ten years' usage) risks of serious side effects are low in women under 35 who are healthy and non-smokers; more regular menstrual periods and less cramping than when a non-pill user; less iron deficiency anemia because menstrual flow is less in quantity and duration; some evidence that Pill may protect against endometrial or ovarian cancer and fibrocystic breast disease.

— **Disadvantages/Contraindications:** increased incidence of bladder and vaginal infections; increased incidence of blood clots (thrombophlebitis, emboli, strokes), cardiovascular and respiratory disease, especially among Pill users who smoke; at least twice the risk of MI as non-Pill users and risk is *greater* than twice as the age, amount of smoking, BP, and/or overweight increases; long-term risks of women who have used Pill more than ten years are still in question but are believed to include atrophy of ovaries, resulting in difficulty resuming normal menstrual periods and achieving normal fertility; higher incidence of cervicitis; higher incidence of breast cancer *when* there is a grandmother/aunt family history of breast cancer.

The Pill should *not* be used by women who have had a stroke, heart attack, anginal chest pains, cancer, blood clots, renal or liver disease, high cholesterol levels, or high blood pressure. The Pill is contraindicated for those with a history of severe migraine headaches, depressions, or diabetes; for those who have a family history of breast cancer; for those who are overweight, over 35, or who are heavy smokers (more than 15 cigarettes per day). Lactating mothers should also avoid taking the Pill.

— Women new to the Pill should have a complete history and physical exam with screening and diagnostic tests (Pap smear, mammogram or Xerography, urine sugar and protein, prothrombin time, hemoglobin and hematocrit counts). Follow-up medical visits on a regular basis are necessary throughout the Pill-taking years to assess physical condition and untoward symptoms.

— **Side Effects:** Those that are relatively minor, transient and to be expected, although annoying, include for some: nausea, headaches, weight gain, sore or tender breasts, and "breakthrough bleeding" (pinkish spotting mid-cycle). These may disappear after a few months adjustment to the hormone level. Some women develop, after 1-2 years, melasma or chloasma (brown patches on face skin similar to "mask" of pregnancy). Use of sun screen lotions helps minimize this. Indications of serious problems should be reported to doctor immediately. These signs include: severe headache, loss of vision, shortness of breath, sudden chest, arm or leg pains and warmth, redness or swelling of calf, thigh, or forearm; persistent vaginal discharge or heavier than usual vaginal bleeding. After the initial adjustment period, if a woman misses a menstrual period, she should find out if she is pregnant before continuing to take Pill in order to reduce possibility of birth defects in the developing fetus.

— **Nursing responsibilities** include responsibility for or assistance with history, physical, and test on initial visit and preliminary patient teaching and counseling. Literature, complete explanations, and opportunities to answer all questions should be provided. Especially important are reminders to report immediately any serious side effects. Written information on what to do when one (or more) pill(s) is missed should be given to each woman to keep readily accessible. "If one Pill is missed, take it with the next day's Pill. If two are missed, take two Pills on each of the next two days and finish series as usual. Use another method of birth control until seven Pills are taken in succession, because disruption such as this can have a rebound effect so the chances of getting pregnant are greater. If three or more Pills are missed, all the remaining Pills in that series should be discarded and a new 21-day cycle should be started 7 days after taking the last Pill. If a period is missed, call your doctor or clinic and be tested for pregnancy."

Drug Trade Names	Ingredients	
Combination Types	Estrogen	Progestin
Brevicon 21 Day		
Brevicon 28 Day (with 7 inert tabs.)	Ethinyl estradiol 0.035 mg.	Norethindrone 0.5 mg.
Demulen -21		
Demulen -28 (with 7 inert tabs.)	Ethinyl estradiol 0.050 mg.	Ethnodiol diacetate 1 mg.
Enovid 5 mg. (20 day)	Mestranol 0.075 mg.	Norethnodrel 5 mg.
Enovid 10 mg.	Mestranol 0.150 mg.	Norethnodrel 10 mg.
Enovid-E (20 day or 21 day)	Mestranol 0.100 mg.	Norethnodrel 2.5 mg.
Loestrin -21 1/20		
Loestrin -Fe 1/20 (7 tabs. brown with ferrous fumarate)	Ethinyl estradiol 0.020 mg.	Norethindrone 1 mg.
Loestrin -21 1.5/30	Ethinyl estradiol 0.030 mg.	Norethindrone 1.5 mg
Lo/Ovral	Ethinyl estradiol 0.030 mg.	Norgestrel 0.3 mg.
Modicon (21 day or 28 day with 7 inert)	Ethinyl estradiol 0.030 mg.	Norethindrone 0.5 mg.
Norinyl 1 + 50 (21 or 28 day with 7 inert)	Mestranol 0.050 mg.	Norethindrone 1 mg.
Norinyl 1 + 80 (21 or 28 day with 7 inert)	Mestranol 0.080 mg.	Norethindrone 1 mg.
Norinyl 2 mg.	Mestranol 0.100 mg.	Norethindrone 2 mg.
Norlestrin 1 mg. (21 or 28 day, 7 inert) (or 28 day with 7 tabs. ferrous fumarate)	Ethinyl estradiol 0.050 mg.	Norethindrone 1 mg.
Ortho-Novum 1/50 (21 or 28 day, 7 inert)	Mestranol 0.050 mg.	Norethindrone 1 mg.
Ortho-Novum 1/80 (21 or 28 day, 7 inert)	Mestranol 0.080 mg.	Norethindrone 1 mg.
Ovcon -35	Ethinyl estradiol 0.035 mg.	Norethindrone 0.4 mg.
Ovcon -50	Ethinyl estradiol 0.050 mg.	Norethindrone 1 mg.
Ovral	Ethinyl estradiol 0.050 mg.	Norgestrel 0.5 mg.
Ovulen (20, 21, or 28 day with 7 inert)	Mestranol 0.100 mg.	Ethnodiol diacetate 1 mg.

Drug	Trade Names	Ingredients

Progestin Only Types | | Estrogen | | Progestin
Micronor | | | | Norethindrone 0.35 mg.
Nor-Q.D. | | | | Norethindrone 0.35 mg.
Ovrette | | | | Norgestrel 0.075 mg.

Recommended References

Can Smokers Take the Pill? and *You and the Pill*, Planned Parenthood Federation of America, Inc., 810 Seventh Ave., New York, NY 10019.
"Oral Contraceptives: How Best To Explain Their Effect to Patients," by Marie Cowart and David Newton. *Nursing 76*, June 1976:44-48.
Physicians' Desk Reference, 35th Ed. Oradell, NJ: Medical Economics Co. 1981.

Drugs: Corticosteroids

GOALS: The patient's disease symptoms are reduced and controlled; the patient takes the medication correctly and safely at the appropriate dosage levels; serious complications and untoward reactions are prevented or controlled.

General Considerations:
— **Types of adrenal corticosteroids** (natural hormones produced by adrenal cortex or synthetic derivatives):
  - glucocorticoids, chiefly cortisone and hydrocortisone that regulate metabolism of CHO, protein and fat;
  - mineralocorticoids, chiefly aldosterone and desoxycorticosterone, which regulate electrolyte and water balance.
  Both are essential to life and must be replaced or supplemented in serious diseases.
— **Therapeutic uses:** often prescribed in a variety of diseases, including pericarditis, dermatitis, collagen skin diseases, rheumatoid arthritis, leukemia, Addison's Disease, bilateral adrenalectomy or post hypophysectomy, asthma, ulcerative colitis, rheumatic fever, severe allergic conditions and serum reactions, certain eye conditions.
— **Pharmacological actions:**
  - reduces inflammation, edema, pain, tenderness, stiffness, pruritis;
  - suppresses lymphatic system, reducing white blood cells;
  - depresses immunoglobulins (antibodies);
  - regulates metabolism and electrolyte balance.
— **Contraindications:** corticosteroids are curative only as replacement therapy in cases of adrenal insufficiency. In other diseases, they must be used cautiously because, while they relieve symptoms, they usually do not affect the cause of the disease. In infectious conditions, for example, they mask the underlying infection, so are usually contraindicated unless — as in some skin conditions — an anti-infective agent is also prescribed. Because corticosteroids promote soduim retention in kidneys and decrease serum calcium and potassium levels as well as affect glucose, protein and fat metabolism, they must be used very cautiously in the presence of hypertension, congestive heart failure, pregnancy, chronic nephritis, renal insufficiency, diabetes mellitus, osteoporosis, and other diseases adversely affected by these actions of corticosteroids. They are also not used for patients with a peptic ulcer history, because corticosteroids undesirably affect the protective gastric mucosa.

— **Treatment** may take the form of: daily replacement therapy (for adrenal insufficiency); alternate day therapy to maintain patients with symptomatic relief of chronic conditions; tapered dosage therapy for ten days or less to treat acute allergic or inflammatory illnesses; inhalation therapy for asthmatics; topical application therapy for skin conditions; and long-acting injections of steroid suspensions (intra-articular, intrasynovial, intrabursal, intradermal, intramuscular).

— **Nursing responsibilities** include:
  - thoroughly understanding corticosteroids: the dosage, administration, action, side & untoward effects and nursing implications for each specific drug (Read the drug literature for the most accurate up-to-date information, since the side effects vary in degree with different synthetic forms of corticosteroids as well as the dosage and administration schedule.);
  - administering each drug precisely as ordered, including questioning and verifying with physician when nursing knowledge and judgment indicates;
  - carefully observing, interviewing patient/family and reporting physiological and psychological responses to drug therapy;
  - conscientiously monitoring patient's vital signs, diet, hygiene, and activities appropriate for corticosteroid therapy (see below nursing implications); and
  - educating patient/family, in collaboration with the doctor, to assume responsibilities of corticosteroid therapy without unduly overwhelming patient with the complexities and undesirable side effects.

Drug Types & Actions	Examples	Side Effects*	Nursing Implications
Natural Glucocorticoids		* N.B. Side effects and nursing implications apply in varying degrees to patients depending on the type of corticosteroid prescribed, the dosage and administration schedule, and the type of disease indications.	
Cortisone Acetate	*Compound E* *Cortone Acetate*		
Hydrocortisone	*Cort-dome, Cortef,* *Cortril, Hydrocortone*	Consult with physician and pharmacist for specific information. *Any* of these side effects and nursing implications can apply to any of the drugs listed.	
Synthetic Glucocorticoids			
Betamethasone	*Celestone*	glycosuria	— check urine BID for glycosuria.

Drug Types & Actions	Examples	Side Effects*	Nursing Implications
Dexamethasone	*Decadron, Deronil, Dexameth, Dexone, Gammacorten, Hexadrol*	voracious appetite excessive thirst	— monitor high-CHO, high-Pro, Lo-Fat diet
Methylprednisolone	*Medrol*	capillary fragility bruisability delayed wound healing	— teach & maintain habits of good hygiene, skin care & foot care
Prednisone	*Delta-Dome, Deltasone, Meticorten, Paracort, Servisone*	growth suppression in children	— check height monthly
Triamcinolone	*Aristocort, Kenacort, Rocinolone*	relief of pain, tenderness, swelling	— see that pt. does not overwork pain-free joints
Natural Mineralocorticoids			
Desoxycorticosterone Acetate	*DOCA Acetate, Percorten Acetate*	alters protective gastric mucosa	— give milk, food, antacids with medications between meals — observe for melena, hematemesis
Synthetic Mineralocorticoids			
FludrocortisoneAcetate	*Florinef Acetate*	abnormal body fat distribution, moon face, acne thrombocytosis	— counsel & assure that changes are reversible — observe & report leg swelling, pain, phlebitis
		mood changes, insomnia, listlessness, depression, euphoria, talkativeness lower seizure threshold	— observe & report all pt. behavior responses — note muscular rigidity, convulsions,

Drug Types & Actions	Examples	Side Effects*	Nursing Implications
			especially in (more susceptible) children
			— seizure precautions
		increased BP sodium retention edema	— check BP twice daily
			— weigh daily
			— offer Low-Na diet
		decrease in serum calcium levels increased calcium & potassium excretion	— offer calcium, potassium and protein rich foods
			— help prevent falls, injuries
		decrease in bone matrix formation anorexia	— keep pt. mobile & physically active
			— offer small feedings several times daily

Discharge Planning and Teaching Outcomes

1) (Patient/Family/Significant Other) Can describe the type of corticosteroids s/he is taking, their use, action, expected and untoward side effects, prescribed dosage, and appropriate, safe, accurate administration.

2) States s/he knows that corticosteroid medication should be taken at same time every day (or every other day) as prescribed. Will keep a written calendar and time record. (Serum hormone levels vary during sleep/awake cycles, being higher in morning and lower in evening. By maintaining a normal daily pattern, untoward effects can be minimized, it is believed).

3) Can tell why corticosteroids must never be stopped abruptly or lapsed for a few days. Has plans for refilling prescriptions well in advance of need, and for carrying a supply in purse or wallet, along with an extra prescription and an identification card giving medication information. (An ID necklace or bracelet is also desirable to wear. ID should be continued for six months to two years post therapy because sudden stress can occur and the patient's own endogenous corticosteroid secretion may still be insufficient to meet body needs.

4) States why s/he must tell dentists, surgeons, psychiatrists or counselors, and emergency room personnel that s/he is taking corticosteroids. (Dosage needs to be increased during biological or psychological stress events).

5) States s/he will take corticosteroid medication with milk, food, or antacid and will try to avoid other ulcer-causing irritants (alcohol, caffeine, aspirin, smoking) during therapy. S/he will report promptly to doctor any burning in esophagus or stomach, or blood in sputum, emesis, or stools.

6) When on a tapering-off schedule, knows to expect fatigue and depression as normal consequences.

7) Knows to report promptly to physician any fever of more than 24 hours, infection, nausea, vomiting, diarrhea, weakness, fatigue, weight loss or gain, dizziness, hypoglycemia or other unusual symptoms or feelings. Knows to report occasions of stress increases, so that dosage can be increased temporarily.

8) Knows to report symptoms of hyperglycemia (increased urination, increased thirst and appetite, fatigue) and fluid/electrolyte imbalance (weight changes of 5 lbs., irregular heart beat, weakness).

9) Knows to watch for falls, because of decreased calcium absorption and susceptibility to osteoporosis.

10) Knows to carefully tend to minor injuries and good skin and foot care because of increased susceptibility to bruising, delayed wound healing, and masked symptoms of infection.

11) When applying topical applications of corticosteroids, knows to avoid air-tight dressings because absorption will be enhanced and side effects more likely to occur.

Recommended References

Physicians' Desk Reference (Current Edition). Oradell, NJ: Medical Economics Co.

"Teaching Patients About Adrenal Corticosteroids," by Pamela Miller Gotch. *The American Journal of Nursing*, January 1981:78-81.

"You Can Minimize the Hazards of Corticosteroids," by David Newton, Arlene Nichols, and Marian Newton. *Nursing 77*, June 1977:26-33.

Drugs: Glaucoma

Goal: The patient's glaucoma symptoms will be reduced and controlled; the patient will recognize side effects and report to physician; the patient will comply with medical regimen.

General Considerations:
- **Caution:** Drugs which increase introcular fluid are *contraindicated:* Mydriatics (Atropine, Scopolomine,) stimulants, or drugs which increase blood pressure.
- Primary open-angle glaucoma has a gradual, insidious onset, and its control depends upon permanent drug therapy (usually combination of miotics to increase outflow of aqueous humor and carbonic anhydrase inhibitors to decrease production of aqueous humor).
- Acute closed-angle glaucoma is an emergency situation in which intraocular pressure increases rapidly; if left untreated, blindness may occur. Treatment with miotic drugs and carbonic anhydrase inhibitors may control intraocular tension in some patients so that surgery is not needed; this treatment may be used before surgery (iridectomy: refer to NCPG #5:10, "The Patient with Glaucoma: Surgical Treatment").
- Secondary glaucoma (following cataract extraction or previous eye disease) is treated by drug therapy.
- **Nursing responsibilities** include knowing actions, side effects, and nursing implications for prescribed drugs; charting patient responses to the drugs, and notifying physician of side effects; and teaching dosage, actions, side-effects and administration of drugs to patient and family prior to discharge. **Advise strict compliance** with prescribed drugs to control symptoms and prevent blindness.

Drug Type & Action	Side Effects	Nursing Implications
Miotics: constrict the pupil *Pilocarpine* drug of choice in glaucoma	Headache, redness of eye & blurred vision when first using miotic; tolerance tends to develop & higher doses become necessary to produce therapeutic effects	Observe for eye irritation & redness; report to physician; advise patient that s/he may have any or all of the side effects when first using miotic or when dose is increased; report to physician if these

Drug Type & Action	Side Effects	Nursing Implications
		discomforts continue after one week; discard solution if clouded or colored; teach pt. to do same.
Carbachol (Doryl)	Same as Pilocarpine	Used if Pilocarpine does not work; be aware of same nursing implications as Pilocarpine.
Phosopholine iodide	Eye irritation; can cause cataracts & blurred vision; danger of respiratory distress during anesthesia because of systemic absorption;	Assess patient for blurred vision & cataracts; report stat; NOTE: *Must* be stopped two weeks before surgery because of systemic absorption & potential danger of respiratory distress during anesthesia.
Floropryl	Vomiting, diarrhea, tenesmus (spasmodic, painful contractions of anal or bladder & sphincter with persistent desire to move bowels or urinate)	NOTE: oil-soluble & long lasting; observe for early signs of nausea, vomiting, diarrhea, tenesmus & report to physician.
Diamox (taken orally)	Gastric distress, shortness of breath, dermatitis, tingling of extremities, acidosis, ureteral stones	Watch closely for side effects & report to physician before continuing medication; used to prepare patients for closed-angle glaucoma surgery; classified as Carbonic Anhydrase Inhibitor; may control intraocular tension so that surgery is not needed.

Drug Type & Action	Side Effects	Nursing Implications
Timolol maleate (Timoptic)	Mild eye irritation; slight blurred vision; may have adverse effects from beta-adrenergic receptor-blocking agents so avoid use with patient with asthma, heart block, heart failure.	Used for primary open-angle glaucoma; does not interfere with visions: assess patient for history or symptoms of asthma (wheezing, dyspnea), heart failure (retention of fluid in lungs & peripheral tissues, dyspnea, cool extremities, fatigue on exertion), heart block (decrease in heart rate & cardiac output); take vital signs Q4H; alert to changes in heart rate & respiration.
Osmotic agents: shrink the gelatinous vitreous humor; reduce fluid.		
Glyrol (U.S.P. Glycerine, 75%) (Taken orally)	Gastric irritation	Used to treat acute closed-angle glaucoma & to prepare for surgery; administer after meal or snack.

Recommended References

"Glaucomas: Diagnosis and Management," by D. Paton and J.A. Craig. *Clinical Symposia*, 28-2, 1976:3-47.
"Screening for Glaucoma," by Heather Boyd-Monk, *Nursing 1979:*42-45.
"Teaching Patients: General Suggestions," *NCP Guide #1:49*, 2nd Ed., Nurseco, 1980.

Hospice-Care Concepts

Definition: Hospice care is an interdisciplinary program of care with the philosophy of providing palliative and supportive services to meet the physical, psychological, social, and spiritual needs of dying persons and their families.

LONG TERM GOAL: The terminally ill person will live meaningfully to the end of life and be free of pain and noxious symptoms. The family and significant others will receive emotional support to help them cope with this crisis.

General Considerations:

— **The goals of hospice** are directed toward six ends: pain control, symptom control, emotional support, family support, spiritual counseling, and bereavement counseling. A multidisciplinary team administers care: physicians, nurses, social workers, psychologists, dietitians, and physiotherapists are examples of health care workers who may make up the team.

— Hospice patients may be cared for in the hospital, convalescent center, or home. The patient is put on the hospice program when the health care team, family, and patient come to the agreement that further treatment will serve no end in effecting a cure. The patient may move in and out of hospice several times; continuity of care for patient and family is extremely important.

— **Treatment:** Unlike traditional care modalities, diagnosis and cure are not appropriate goals for the terminally ill; palliative care is prescribed. Palliative care is defined as those measures that are designed to control symptoms and promote comfort. Palliative measures that may be prescribed are those that control pain, nausea and vomiting, shortness of breath, diarrhea,or any other noxious stimuli

— The family, as well as the patient, is considered to be part of the client unit of care and also receives nursing assessment and emotional support. Their contact with the patient is recognized as important to the family unit and is encouraged. If on a home-care hospice plan, there must be a family member who is able to be the primary care giver. Some experts feel that the home setting is ideal; most patients agree.

— **Nursing responsibilities:** As a member of the team, the nurse does assessments, makes recommendations, and intervenes with the patient and family:

1) **Pain control.** Ideally, oral analgesics are desired. If the patient is unable to swallow or if uncontrollable nausea is present, parenteral analgesics are acceptable. Analgesics most helpful for intractable pain are morphine and methadone. Both can be administered in liquid form; oral dosages must be given up to 3-6 times the amount administered intramuscularly to

be effective. Compared to morphine, methadone is more readily absorbed orally, has a longer half-life, and thus may be more effective. However, it sometimes takes 24-36 hours to be effective. An antiemetic, such as compazine, is also frequently included. Typical dosage for an adult is 10 mg methadone or 20 mg of morphine in solution, p.o. every 3 to 4 hours. Medication is never given on a PRN schedule but is administered around the clock, awakening the patient at night so that blood levels remain constant. Patients who receive morphine may, initially, be drowsy or sleep around the clock for 24-36 hours but then become alert. The dosage is decreased for those patients who do not become alert after 36 hours. Drug tolerance reportedly is rare. Patients' need for more medication is directly related to the progression of the disease process; the possibility of addiction is not an issue with a dying person and under-medication is cruel and unnecessary. Respiratory depression is reported to cause few problems although this is a concern to health care professionals. If pain is due to muscular, skeletal, or joint pathology, aspirin may be indicated. Other pathology with specific analgesic agents should be treated appropriately, with or without a narcotic elixir as is indicated by patient need.

2) **Symptom control:** In addition to controlling pain, other symptoms should be eliminated:

- *GI Symptoms:* Patients who are on analgesics should be observed for decreased large bowel function; a stool softener may be indicated. Nausea and diarrhea are other distressing symptoms to be controlled.
- *Nutrition and Hydration:* Fluids should be encouraged as tolerated; terminally-ill patients are prone to dehydration. Nourishment may be enhanced with a soft diet or anything that sounds palatable to the patient; foods prepared by family members may be tolerated best. Assess for urinary incontinence and report to physician.
- *Movement:* Comfort can be promoted by regular turning of patients at least every hour. Complete range of motion (ROM) exercises should be done four times a day, either actively or passively (see NCPG #1:47, "ROM Exercises"). Patients should be encouraged to be as active as they can; ambulating, sitting in a chair, turning, moving all extremities, or being turned and moved. Each patient has an individual capability for exercise and movement. Persons who are free of pain and symptoms are more likely to want to move about.
- *Skin Integrity:* Attention to the skin is crucial for comfort since ill patients do not have optimal nutrition and exercise. Frequent turning and movements change soft tissue pressure points and increase speed of circulation. Baths, lotions, back rubs, and gentle massage contribute to patient comfort. Edema causes discomfort and calls for special, gentle handling. Assist patient with oral hygiene after meals and PRN; use mouth swabs and soft tooth brush.

3) **Emotional support:** Dying patients have need for personal contact and to be involved in the mainstream of life. Each

individual is unique and the nurse should visit patient and family often in order to develop a trusting relationship. Encourage the patient to talk about anything that s/he wishes; be a good listener; find mutual interests to discuss. Do not avoid topics of conversation because it makes you uncomfortable. Encourage family members to meet the family members of other patients in the hospice; they will offer a great deal of support to each other. Encourage hobbies, crafts, and interests as tolerated. Children and pets provide a great sense of enjoyment and enrichment. Touch and non-verbal contact have increased meaning to the dying patient.

4) **Family Support:** Families need time and attention of hospice team members just like the patient does. Family members need to talk about their concerns, fears, anger, frustrations, and feelings of loss over their loved one. Allow time to listen to family members and convey to them that you understand. Sharing your feelings is appropriate, too. Answer their questions directly and simply. Encourage family members to engage in some pleasurable activity that does not involve the patient to provide a break for them. The services of child care, housekeeping, patient-sitting, or transportation may be indicated to help the family.

5) **Spiritual Counseling:** Patients and families may have the need for clergy or pastoral care. Assist them to obtain services of a minister or rabbi PRN. In addition, they will want to talk about and consider the positive aspects of their lives and the meaning of life and death. Be available and be an attentive listener.

6) **Bereavement Counseling:** To die and to lose a loved one is at best a difficult task. Talk with your patients and families about their feelings; listen to what they say. Reassure them that their feelings are valid and expected. The completion of the grieving process varies in length for different people; one to two years is usually cited as the time needed. The hospice team stays in contact with the family during this time since the nurse has been closely involved with the family during the care of deceased. The nurse has grief work to do too, since nurses also experience a feeling of loss with the death of their parents. During this time the family adjusts to the loss of their family member, and to life without that person. Tasks of living are taken up and directed towards self fulfillment as was the case before the illness and death of the loved one. See NCP Guide #1:31, "Responses to Loss: The Grief and Mourning Process."

Discharge Planning and Teaching Objectives/Outcomes

1) (Patient/Family/Significant Other) Has knowledge of prognosis, diagnosis, plan of care.
2) Has a supply of medications, knows how and when to administer them, and how to get refills when patient is home. Can describe symptoms and drug side effects that are to be reported to physician.
3) Knows how to help patient with activities of daily living and carry out treatments.

4) Can identify community and hospice support contacts; has names and telephone numbers to call for help.

Recommended References

"Dealing with Impending Death." *NCP Guide #1:27,* 2nd Ed., Nurseco, 1980.

"Four Models of Hospice Care," by R. Dellabough, *Hospital Forum,* January/February 1980:6-7.

"Hospice Comes of Age," by P. Stack. *Nursing Times,* June 12, 1980:1034.

"Hospice: Enabling a Patient to Die at Home," by S.V. Dobihal. *The American Journal of Nursing.* August 1980:1448-1451.

"Hospital Care for the Terminally Ill: A Model Program," by D.R. Longo and K. Darr. *Hospital Progress,* March 1978:62-65.

"Pain Relief for Cancer Patients," by A.S. Valentine et al. *The American Journal of Nursing,* December 1978:2054-2056.

"Range of Motion Exercises." *NCP Guide #1:47,* 2nd Ed., Nurseco, 1980.

"Responses to Loss: The Grief and Mourning Process." *NCP Guide #1:31,* 2nd Ed., Nurseco, 1980.

"Standards for Hospice Address Definition and Quality Concerns," by C.B. Treham. *Hospital Forum,* January/February 1980:16-17.

Nasogastric Intubation: General Principles

Goal: The patient has a nasogastric (or gastrointestinal) tube inserted with safety, privacy, and a minimum of discomfort.

General Considerations:
— **Purpose and indications:** nasogastric or gastrointestinal intubation is used for:
1) *decompression,* to keep cavity empty of fluids and gas for postoperative comfort, prevention of vomiting, and relief of consequences of obstruction and paralytic ileus, as well as to ease tension on suture line;
2) *lavage,* to remove toxic agents;
3) *gavage,* to maintain nutrition or to administer medications; and
4) *analysis* of stomach fluids or cells and the assessment, detection, and treatment of bleeding in the gastrointestinal tract.
— **Types of tubes:** sizes range from 6-18 French; older tubes are made of rubber or hard polyvinyl chloride, newer tubes are made of silicone rubber or softer polyurethane. Short stomach tubes (nasogastric) include:
- *Levin,* a single lumen traditional tube with several drainage openings near the distal tip;
- *Salem Sump,* a double lumen tube within a tube that provides atmospheric air along the outer suction tube so that suction force and mucosal damage are lessened;
- *Blakemore-Sengstaken,* a triple lumen double balloon (esophageal and gastric) tube used to treat esophageal or upper gastric bleeding from varices;
- *Dobbhoff,* an enteric feeding tube of polyurethane with a mercury weight at the distal end;
- *Keofeed* tube, a soft silicone rubber tube with a mercury weight at the distal end;
- *Med Pro,* a silicone rubber tube enclosed in a stiff polyvinyl chloride tube that facilitates passage and then is removed, leaving the smaller tube in place;
— Longer intestinal tubes (gastrointestinal) include:
- *Harris and Cantor,* single lumen tubes with bags at the distal end that are filled with mercury before use;
- *Miller-Abbott,* a double lumen tube: one outlet used for drainage and one within the balloon at the end, which is filled with air or mercury. The proximal end of this outlet is carefully tied off and clearly marked, and the drainage outlet is attached to suction;
- *Abbot-Dawson,* a double lumen tube, one ending about eight inches beyond the drainage lumen. The more distal lumen has a metal bulb attached to facilitate passage by gravity and peristalisis.

- **Complications and side effects:**
    1) traumatic gastric ulcers may result from excessive negative suction pressure that pulls mucosa into tube lumen;
    2) acute parotitis related to poor oral hygiene and debilitated condition;
    3) esophagitis, pharyngitis, and laryngitis from tubes in place several days;
    4) esophageal or gastric bleeding associated with use of larger tubes (#14 and up) or with stress, mucosal irritation, cortisone levels, etc;
    5) aspiration pneumonia from increased secretions along tube's pathway; and
    6) severe dehydration and electrolyte imbalance related to constant gastric suction.
- **Measurement for intubation:** based on studies done during autopsy, findings indicate recommended distance for insertion of the tube to a proper distance of 1-10 cm. beyond the lower esophageal sphincter (LES) is:
    for infants: the length equal to the distance from the tip of the nose to the ear lobe, and to a point midway between the tip of the xiphoid and the umbilicus; and
    for adults: the nose-ear-xiphoid tip (NEX) measurement is accurate for approximately 70% of patients; for increased accuracy, measure 50 cm. on the tube, then measure the NEX distance on the tube, then mark the stopping place on the tube as halfway between these two points. Insertion of the tube this distance will place it properly, less than 12 cm. beyond the LES into the fundus of stomach in most patients (90%).

Nursing Actions and General Principles of Tube Insertion:
1) Provide sufficient light, working space and privacy so that nurse and patient can work together comfortably. Explain tube's purpose as well as procedure for passage after determining what the patient knows and wishes to know. Arrange a "stop" signal that patient can use to direct you to pause a moment during passage of tube.
2) Arrange all necessary equipment and supplies in a readily accessible place to save time and energy. Efficiency helps maintain the patient's confidence in the nurse's competence. Suggested items include:
    — towel drape for patient, facial tissues;
    — glass of drinking water with flexible straw (ice chips may be used but are not recommended);
    — basin of warm water or ice (too soft or limp tubes are stiffened by placing in ice for 15-20 minutes; too stiff plastic tubes can be softened for curling and ease of passage by placing in warm water for a few minutes prior to use);
    — tube ordered by doctor, Hoffman clamp, suction apparatus, asepto syringe;

— *water-soluble* lubricant (No mineral oil!), masking tape or hypoallergenic tape and a safety pin.

3) Have the conscious patient sit in a high Fowler's position. Drape chest with towel. Give patient tissue to hold in one hand (for tearing eyes) and the glass of water with straw in other hand.

4) Measure distance of tube insertion (see above) for placement in stomach and mark tube with a piece of tape.

5) Liberally lubricate entire length of tube to "passage-stop" mark. (Some people lubricate only first 3-4 inches, but experience has shown more effective, less irritating passage with generous lubrication.)

6) Using gentle, persistent pressure insert lubricated tube into one nostril to posterior pharyngeal wall. Patient's head should not be hyperextended, but flexed so that swallowing is facilitated. If the tube will not move downward, even with slight inward rotation and downward pressure, remove tube and try other nostril. (Passage through mouth is used when necessary but avoided when possible; take precaution to remove dentures.) When tube reaches pharynx have patient lean forward and drink sips of water (or repeatedly swallow air), continually swallowing so that trachea will close, gag reflex can be suppressed, and passage of tube facilitated through esophagus. Keep telling patient how well s/he is doing and how nearly finished you are with insertion. Keep reminding patient to swallow.

If patient is unconscious, turn patient on right side. Place an airway in mouth to depress tongue. Advance tube between patient's breaths and stroke throat and neck to help swallowing and passage of tube. Turn patient to left side after aspiration of stomach contents with syringe.

Remove tube quickly if patient chokes, turns blue, or has difficulty breathing. Otherwise, continue advancement of tube to predetermined mark.

7) Ascertain placement by aspirating stomach contents with a syringe. Advance or withdraw tube until return flow is evident. Tube may be curled and still need to straighten and enter the stomach sphincter. Turn patient to left side so that stomach contents can move into the greater curvature of stomach and be more easily reached. Remove syringe and clamp tube, temporarily.

8) After cleansing cheek skin with alcohol or acetone, tape nasogastric tube to skin and secure. Attach proximal end of tube to low pressure intermittent suction. If tube feedings are ordered, see NCPG #5:50, "Tube Feedings: General Principles."

Gastrointestinal tubes are not taped or secured, but coiled loosely near patient's head. The tube is advanced 2-4 inches every 1-2 hours as ordered by the physician. The patient's position is changed periodically to facilitate natural advancement of tube into the small intestine. X-rays are ordered to confirm placement.

9) Record accurately amount and type of suction drainage, irrigation solutions used, and liquid tube feedings and medications.

10) Chart tube insertion procedure, patient response, and periodic function of tube (patency, drainage, irrigations, etc.).

On-going Care and Removal:

1) Provide regular mouth care at least Q4H. Have patient brush teeth and massage gums. Gum chewing or sucking on hard candies is sometimes permitted and encouraged. Gargles and mouth washes with warm saline should be done three times daily. Antiseptic and anesthetic solutions, sprays or lozenges may be prescribed for sore throat. Use cream or ointment for lips and nose to counteract dryness and irritation.

2) To remove tube safely, have patient sit upright. Drape with towel across chest. Give patient a tissue to hold. Irrigate tube with a small amount of saline or tap water. Clamp tube; ask patient to hold breath, then remove tube slowly (not too slowly!), gently and steadily, placing it in towel and covering it from the patient's sight. Record appropriate observations.

Recommended References

"Ensuring Safer Stomach Suctioning with the Salem Sump Tube," by Edwina McConnell. *Nursing 77*, September 1977:54-57.

"New Approach to Measuring Adult Nasogastric Tubes for Insertion," by Robert Hanson. *The American Journal of Nursing*, July 1980:1334-1335.

"Taking the Trauma out of Nasogastric Intubation," by Cecilia Volden, Jacquelyn Grinde, and David Carl. *Nursing 80*, September 1980:64-67.

"Ten Problems with Nasogastric Tubes ... And How to Solve Them," by Edwina McConnell. *Nursing 79*, April 1979:78-81.

"Tube Feedings: General Principles," *NCP Guide #5:50*, Nurseco, 1981.

"Update: Nasogastric Tube Feeding," by Barbara Griggs and Mary Hoppe. *The American Journal of Nursing*, March 1979:481-483.

Problem Solving

"Feed a man a fish and he will eat for a night,
Teach a man how to fish and he will eat for the rest of his life."
—*Anonymous*

Definition: A systematic method of reasoning or organizing data in order to find useful and effective alternative ways to cope with a situation, need, or concern that constitutes a problem.

LONG TERM GOAL: The patient/client/staff member will learn and demonstrate the steps and methods of problem solving; the patient/client/staff member will demonstrate increased ability to solve problem.

General Considerations:

— Effective problem solving is essential to mental health and is a learned behavior; with practice, the learner can improve problem-solving ability; problem solving can be done alone, with one other, or in a group.

— Behaviors that may indicate a need for problem solving include:

- physical discomfort
- powerlessness
- shame or stigma
- passivity
- incompetence in coping with ADL (activities of daily living)

- conflict
- emotional threat
- hopelessness
- increased stress
- non-assertion
- distorted reality testing

- anxiety
- low self-esteem
- frustration
- guilt
- immaturity
- aggression

— **Components** of problem solving are: awareness of problem area, problem definition, data collection and analysis, formulation of alternative solutions, discussion of possible consequences, selection of best alternative, implementation of trial run, evaluation, and summary.

— **Nursing responsibilities** include a knowledge of problem-solving methods and assessment of patient/client/staff members for unresolved problems that require nursing intervention.

Specific Considerations, Potential Patient Outcomes, and Nursing Actions:

1) Awareness of the Problem Area

The patient/client/staff member will see, hear, feel, or experience awareness of specific situation or problem area:
— focus on situation, need or concern; ask person to recall & describe details, including feelings & issues, what was seen & heard, who was involved, when & how event occurred;
— know that awareness is the first step of change; listen & explore without giving advice or jumping to conclusions.

2) Problem Definition

The problem(s) will be identified and defined; goals/objectives/expected outcomes will be specified:
— define needs & goals/objectives/expected outcomes; set priorities in terms of most pressing problems;
— identify issues & different aspects involved; separate complex problems into subgroups;
— determine what creates the problem by asking: "Why is it a problem? Who is affected by this? Who else is involved? Who else could be involved in problem solving? Why am I motivated to change the situation?"
— identify who, what, when, where & which; ask open-ended questions, i.e., "How do you manage _____?" "What is it about this situation that concerns you?"

3) Data Collection and Analysis

Data will be collected, organized, and analyzed in an appropriate way:
— decide on a method to collect data which is relevant to the situation (e.g., literature search; create data collection tool to be used to interview in person, by mail, or by telephone survey); problem solving group may be created to bring together individuals with similar problem to share information & offer group support, encouragement;
— organize & classify data, using outline or numbering method; large file cards or computer system may be helpful;
— validate findings with other persons; clarify issues; identify gaps or discrepancies in information;
— analyze data by discussion, comparing & contrasting issues & information;
— interpretation of data involves making a relationship between facts, using the process of induction or deduction to form a conclusion; identify causes of problem & influencing factors.

4) Alternative Solutions

Alternative solutions will be formulated and discussed with consideration of possible consequences:
— formulate tentative alternative solutions, using data analysis & conclusions; consider all possible courses of action; list each as a possible solution;
— discuss each alternative & identify its possible consequences, including pros & cons, strengths & weaknesses; role play alternatives, paying attention to feelings & physiologic responses;
— be aware of person's attitudes, values, & feelings which influence determination of pros & cons;

— assess for lack of knowledge or experience to initiate alternative; health teach as needed in assertiveness, communication skills, interpersonal relationship skills.

5) Trial Run and Evaluation

An alternative solution will be chosen and a trial run will be implemented and evaluated:

— choose one possible solution that seems most appropriate; plan and initiate trial run; complex plans should be broken down into small steps;

— identify specific actions to be taken; assess knowledge & skills needed to obtain PRN; estimate time needed & anticipate factors that may facilitate or hinder the action;

— know that trial runs usually have to be modified or revised; continue collecting data to revise or modify as needed;

— be flexible & open-minded; if the alternative is not satisfactory, try another one. *There are always other alternatives!* You may find that you need to start back at the first or second step with awareness & redefinition of the problem;

— evaluate effectiveness of alternative solution in relation to the previously set goals and objectives.

6) Summary

The problem-solving method will be summarized, including problem-solving process and content; anticipatory guidance will be offered to cope with next problem:

— summarize the problem-solving process, using the problem-solving components & the specific content; this may be done verbally or with charts, graphs, audio visuals, or written reports may be created to share the conclusion or results with others;

— identify future situations which may be potential problem areas & use anticipatory guidance to apply conclusions, alternative solutions, or problem-solving methods to these situations; give positive reinforcement for ability to apply new knowledge to potential problem situations;

— recognize & give verbal & non-verbal positive reinforcement for willingness to learn & use problem-solving methods & for demonstrations of increased ability to problem solve.

Recommended References

"Behavior Modification." *NCP Guide #5:37*, Nurseco, 1981.

"The Liaison Nurse: Centralizing Problem-Solving," by B.M. LeClear. *Supervisor Nurse*, March 1980:42–43.

"Meeting the Challenge of Fistulas and Draining Wounds," by Sr. V. Taylor. *Nursing '80*, June 1980:45–51.

"Nursing Decisions . . . Stroke!" by M.J. Stillman. *RN*, November 1979:49–56.

"The Patient Experiencing Guilt." *NCP Guide #5:31*, Nurseco, 1981.

"The Patient Experiencing a Threat to Self-Esteem." *NCP Guide #5:32*, Nurseco, 1981.

"The Patient Experiencing Powerlessness." *NCP Guide #5:34,* Nurseco, 1981.
"The Patient Experiencing Shame/Embarrassment." *NCP Guide #5:35,* Nurseco, 1981.
"Problem-Oriented Charting." *NCP Guide #2:49,* 2nd Ed., Nurseco, 1980.
"Suggestions for Interviewing." *NCP Guide #1:44,* 2nd Ed., Nurseco, 1980.

Radiation Therapy: General Principles

Definition: Radiation therapy is treatment of a person with an ionizing radioactive substance or with roentgen rays for the purpose of destroying malignant cells or to make them incapable of further cell division.

LONG TERM GOAL: The patient will respond therapeutically with maximum benefits to radiation therapy and will experience reduced pain, symptomatic relief, minimum side effects and restoration of confidence; the patient will accept/adapt to bio-psycho-social aspects of cancer diagnosis with recommended radiation treatment and continuing care.

General Considerations:

— Fifty to sixty per cent of all cancer patients receive radiation therapy at some stage of their disease. Some will experience a cure; others, an extension and improvement in quality of life.

— **Radiation therapy may be administered by** ingestion, injection, isotope implantaion, or, externally, with kilovoltage (thousands of electron volts, KeV) or megavoltage (millions of electron volts, MeV) machines. Examples of machines commonly in use include the linear accelerator, the cobalt 60 teletherapy machine, the Van de Graff Generator and the betatron. The type of energy and the depth of penetration required by the tumor determine the machine to be used. Kilovoltage machines produce a soft x-ray of low penetration and quickly-absorbed energy. They are used for superficial lesions such as skin, breast, or parotid tumors. Megavoltage machines can deliver a sharper beam of deeper penetration (10 cm) thus "sparing" the skin and concentrating its energy on the tumor target.

— **Radiation therapy may be used as** a single, curative modality when disease is localized, as in cervical cancer, skin cancer, or primary Hodgkin's Disease; or as a synergistic combination modality for palliative as well as curative purposes in conditions with circulating cancer cells, such as lymphocytic leukemia or breast cancer with metastases. Total Body Irradiation (TBI) is the exposure of the entire body to a massive dose of gamma radiation in order to penetrate sites more resistant to antineoplastic therapy.

— **Radiation symbol** is the universal sign indicating radioactive materials are being stored or used in the area. The warning sign is a purple propeller on a yellow field. The radiation department provides these for use where needed in the nursing units.

— **Radiation reaction & side effects:** An effort is made to deliver a maximum dose to the tumor with a minimum dose to surrounding healthy tissue. Shielding of healthy organs is routine, and, as mentioned above, newer MeV machines have skin-sparing assets. Despite precautions, some normal cells and tissues may receive acute damage accounting for moderate to severely distressing side effects. Side effects vary depending on the part of body irradiated as well as the dose, rate, time-rate fractionation, and total applied dose. After-effects may be acute, intermediate, or late (months to years post treatment) depending on the extent and type of cells and tissue damaged. Acute reactions occur during treatment, are temporary and controllable. An example is *Radiation Syndrome* (also known as Radiation Sickness), a relatively mild illness manifested by headache, anorexia, nausea, vomiting, and diarrhea. Late reactions, on the other hand, are serious and irreversible. These include growth retardation, sterility, cataracts, and liver or kidney damage.

— **Gastrointestinal reactions and nutritional problems** are caused by physiological response to radiation treatments, by emotional stress, and/or by disease effects on GI tract. When patient has had a previous weight loss, surgery, and/or chemotherapy, nutritional problems are compounded. Irradiation of the head and neck can cause highly radiosensitive oral mucous membranes to become lacerated and infection-prone. Local mucositis, buccal inflammation, sore throat, decreased salivation (thick, sticky, and acid saliva) and damage to blood vessels feeding the jaws may occur. There is increased susceptibility to cavities (extending for years post treatment). Symptoms leading to malnutrition include anorexia, nausea, vomiting, diarrhea, and difficulty swallowing. Common are changes in taste such as deteriorated taste perceptions (hypogeusesthesia) or perverted taste sensations (dysgeusia) with complaints of food tasting rancid, salty, bitter, metallic, or spoiled. Nursing measures and dietary modifications are essential (see below). Sometimes parenteral hyperalimentation or tube feedings become necessary when malnutrition, edema, and negative nitrogen balance are evident.

— **Skin reactions** are influenced not only by the area of exposure and amount of dosage as mentioned earlier, but also by the patient's skin quality and care, sensitivity to irritation, and the presence of infection or previous injury. Radiodermatitis reactions include rashes, erythema, dryness, itchiness, progressive blistering and wet desquamation (sloughing of skin surface).

— **Cardiopulmonary reactions:** Irradiation of the chest may produce pneumonitis (persistent hacking cough, fever, dyspnea, and weakness). Pericarditis may occur up to a year after treatment; symptoms include chest pain and friction rub. Both respond to treatment. These complications are more common when patient has a pulmonary infection, concurrent pulmonary disease, or toxic reaction to chemotherapy.

— **Other radiation reactions** include alopecia (hairs grows back in several months), increased intracranial pressure, a drop in blood count, and bone marrow depression. Transfusions and bone marrow transplants are often necessary after total body irradiation.

— **Nursing responsibilities** for patients receiving radiation therapy include:

  (1) assessment of patient/family needs re: acceptance and readiness to participate positively in prescribed therapy;

(2) orientation, counseling, and teaching activities reinforcing physicians explanations and directions re: treatment aims, expected effects, procedures, and patient behaviors necessary for maximum therapeutic benefit and successful coping with side effects;

(3) planning and implementation of care for observed side effects of radiation;

(4) implementation of safety precautions for personnel, patients, family, and visitors when patient is receiving internal radiation therapy (refer to NCPG #5:16, "The Patient with Radiation Implant/GYN"); and

(5) referrals to nursing home, community health agency, other clinics and social services PRN.

Specific Considerations, Potential Patient Outcomes, and Nursing Actions:

1) Patient/ Family Teaching

The patient/family can explain the proposed radiation treatment plan and aims; the patient/family can tell what side effects may occur and how they can cope successfully with these; the patient/family expresses confidence and optimistic attitudes re: ability to cooperate with treatment regimen and to be mutually supportive:

— assess knowledge of radiation therapy, treatment plan for pt., expected & possible side effects, role in cooperating with treatment & care regimen;

— provide information booklet from radiation dept., if available; arrange tour of radiation dept. & introductions to personnel; utilize group teaching sessions with other pts. & families when deemed advantageous; provide time for questions, taking time to find out answers you do not know; include in topics: the coldness of room, the noisiness of big machines, the waiting time for setting up treatments, the length of treatments, the lonely, frightening feelings of isolation, the observation method (TV monitior or viewing window), the two-way voice communication that can be used;

— provide written instructions (if pt. is on an out-pt. basis) on skin care, dietary modifications, appt. times for treatments, phone numbers to call for information, help, & medications.

2) Nutrition

The patient's ability to eat is restored and optimal nutrition is maintained:

— arrange for consultation with dietician so that individual pt. preferences can be considered;

— know that sample diets can be obtained from local American Cancer Society;

— weigh daily;

— give vitamin & mineral supplements prescribed;

— give pain relief & antiemetic medications approximately two hours before mealtimes;

- arrange for family or friends to be present during meals, since encouragement & companionship help to stimulate appetite & increase amt. eaten;
- arrange for larger meals when anorexia & nausea are least (usually early AM); otherwise plan several small meals & feedings daily;
- offer bland, high-protein foods such as cream cheese, cottage cheese, gelatin salad with fruit, ice cream, puddings, & milkshakes;
- between meals, serve cold high-protein, high-caloric commercial supplements;
- know that cold, bland foods can be used to numb & relieve painful mouths; avoid serving hot foods that aggravate mouth soreness; avoid coffee, tea, alcoholic & carbonated beverages that will cause irritation; know that cooked fruits may be tolerated but citrus or acid types will be rejected when buccal inflamation worsens; puree coarse foods & strain PRN;
- offer liquid antacids to neutralize oral acidity & lessen cavity proneness;
- provide caries-prevention & prophylactic oral hygiene in the form of daily flossing, Water Pik irrigations, weekly fluoride mouth washes, & gentle cleansing of teeth & mouth; to provide relief of soreness, use ice chips, xylocaine mouth washes & power spray rinsing with solutions of H_2O_2 (peroxide) & NS; be careful of friable buccal membranes;
- when ability to salivate is lessened, making swallowing difficult, try gravies & sauces on soft foods to help; otherwise, tube feedings may be necessary when weight loss becomes severe; see NCPG #5:50, "Tube Feedings: General Principles;"
- for diarrhea & bowel malabsorption (related to radiation-induced small bowel enteritis), offer low-residue, low-lactose foods; serve liquid feedings that are half-strength, flavored, & very cold; urge pt. to sip slowly to reduce cramping & to enhance absorption; give antidiarrheic medications (such as Lomotil or Kaopectate,) as prescribed.

3) Skin Protection

The patient's skin is protected from excessive damage, is soothed and healed:
- know & explain to pt. that indelible dye markings, delineating areas to be treated or blocked out of field, will be made on skin of appropriate body region; tell pt. that these must not be removed or altered;
- see that skin in radiation area is only rinsed gently with tepid water (no soap is permitted except sometimes a

bland Neutrogena-type); no rubbing is allowed; nothing is applied to skin without specific written permission of attending radiologist/oncologist;
- *with orders,* rinse damaged skin with hydrogen peroxide & saline mixture; pat dry; apply cornstarch for itching or, for dryness use bland ointment such as A & D Ointment; antibiotic or hydrocortisone ointment may be prescribed for severe redness, blistering, or infection;
- observe & report redness, tautness, itching, dryness, blistering, & desquamation;
- for wet-draining areas, use non-adhering dressings & tubular stretch bandages with non-allergenic tape;
- teach pt. to avoid sun or heat applications for several years following treatment; teach pt. to avoid constricting clothes that rub or irritate & to be careful of injuries to skin that may be slow healing.

Recommended References

"Nursing Care During Total Body Irradiation." by Claudette G. Varricchio. *The American Journal of Nursing*, August 1977:1314-1317.

"Nutritional Problems in Radiotherapy Patients," by James C. Rose. *The American Journal of Nursing*, July 1978:1194-1106.

"The Patient On Radiation Therapy," by Claudette G. Varricchio. *The American Journal of Nursing*, February 1981:334-337.

"The Patient with Radiation Implant/GYN." *NCP Guide #5:16*, Nurseco, 1981.

"Radiation Therapy: How You Can Help," by Carolyn St. John Elliott. *The American Journal of Nursing*, September 1976:34-41.

"Planning Care For the Patient Receiving External Radiation," by Patricia Paul Delly and Cynthia Tinsley. *The American Journal of Nursing*, February 1981:338-342.

"Tube Feedings: General Principles." *NCP Guide #5:50*, Nurseco, 1981.

Stress Management

Definition: *Stress* is a generalized, non-specific response of the body to any demand or change, whether positive or negative. *Stressors* are the demands or changes and may be real or anticipated. *Distress* is damaging or unpleasant stress.

GOAL: The patient will maintain homeostasis or optimal adaptive coping by preventing, or recognizing promptly, excessive levels of stress and by utilizing effective measures to manage it.

General Considerations:
— The human body constantly interacts with the environment to maintain physiological and psychosocial homeostasis (optimal adaptive coping).
— **The stress syndrome** is described by Hans Selye as the General Adaptation Syndrome (or GAS). It consists of three stages: the alarm stage, the resistance stage, and the exhaustion stage:
  1) *The alarm stage* is the initial response of the body to stressors. It serves to protect the body from events that threaten homeostasis. Responses are generalized throughout the body and include increased heart rate and respiration, elevation in blood sugar level, increase in perspiration, dilated pupils, slowed digestion, increased activity and alertness, constriction of the blood vessels of the skin, and increased clotting ability of the blood.
  2) *The resistance stage:* the body's defenses, both physiological and psychological, are mobilized to resist the stress. The body adapts to the stress as best it can and repairs any damage resulting from it. When resistance is successful, the characteristic responses of the alarm stage virtually disappear.
  3) *The exhaustion stage* occurs when the body's finite store of adaptive energy is used up (usually after a prolonged period of time); the body's defenses are insufficient to cope with the stress and stressors. If this stage continues long enough, the individual may develop one of the "diseases of stress" such as migraine or tension headaches, hypertension, heart irregularity, peptic ulcer, or others. Continued exposure to stressors during this stage causes the body to run out of adaptive energy, and may even stop functioning. Chronic stress causes chronic disease and can lower the body's resistance to infectious disease.
— **Stress is an ongoing part of life;** a certain amount of stress is essential for survival and allows the individual to function at an alert, efficient level—excessive levels are unhealthful. Each person has a unique optimal level of stress and can learn

to cope with stress adaptively.
- **Distress** causes the body to constantly readjust or adapt. Signs of distress include:

- irritability
- emotional tension
- emotional instability
- impulsive behavior
- inability to concentrate
- chronic fatigue
- accident proneness

- sweating
- frequent urination
- diarrhea or constipation
- insomnia
- decrease or increase of appetite
- alcohol and drug abuse
- neurotic or psychotic behaviors

- increased smoking
- nightmares
- headache
- pain in neck or back
- grinding of teeth
- stuttering
- sexual problems

- **Nursing responsibilities** include assessing for signs of distress and maladaptive responses to change, identifying stressors and stage of stress syndrome, and prescribing interventions to promote homeostasis and adaptive coping with stress and stressors. Patient education is vital to promote and maintain optimal adaptive coping.

General Suggestions for Managing Stress Adaptively:
1) **Exercise** daily. Physical activity allows an outlet for mental stress as well as developing flexibility, muscular strength and endurance, and increasing efficiency of body system functioning. Walking, running, dancing, swimming, gardening, participating in sports or body movement exercises, and yoga are examples of methods to reduce stress through exercise. Many community gyms, health clubs, and YMCAs have regular group exercise programs that are fun and enjoyable as well as healthy. Consult personal physician for contraindications to exercise program.
2) **Develop alternative ways to relax.** Choose activities you really enjoy and plan to devote at least an hour a day pursuing them. Allow yourself to explore creative activities such as drawing, pottery, carpentry, writing, musical activities, or photography; let yourself read a good book, watch the sunset, listen to music, take a bubble bath, or cultivate the fine art of short naps. Let yourself remember ways you have relaxed in the past (sports, music) and experience these old ways again. Try something new and different; check out various community activities available through recreation departments, adult education programs, community colleges.
3) **Learn mental exercises** to create a sense of peace and tranquility and to relax muscles. Examples include:
   - *Progressive relaxation:* concentrate on relaxing successive sets of muscles from the tips of your toes to the top of your head; this may include tightening one set of muscles and then letting go of the muscles to a count of six. For example, "I'm

holding tight the muscles in my hand and arm — 1, 2, 3, 4, 5, 6: I'm letting go of the muscles in my hand and arm — 1, 2, 3, 4, 5, 6, with the holding lasting for 15-30 seconds and the letting go lasting an equal amount of time. An alternative way to do progressive relaxation is to focus by saying, "My feet are becoming relaxed and warm; my ankles are becoming relaxed and warm," and progressivily focusing on each successive part of the body.

- *Autogenic training exercises:* repeat verbal formulas with passive concentration and relaxed posture; examples: "My body is becoming warm and relaxed. I am beginning to feel quiet and relaxed. My right arm is warm and relaxed. My heart beat is calm and regular. My lungs breathe for me. My forehead is cool. My jaw is relaxed and easy."
- *Imagery:* use your imagination to daydream, to reminisce, or to remember positive experiences. Focus on your favorite vacation spot and let yourself see, hear, smell, taste, and feel the breeze of that relaxed, pleasurable experience. Concentrate on a beautiful drawing or photograph; let yourself drift off in your imagination to become part of the picture. Listen to music and allow yourself to imagine scenes and pleasurable experiences that the music evokes. Imagine yourself as healthy, effective, graceful, flexible, relaxed . . . whatever you would like to be; be aware of negative thoughts or images, and replace them with positive ones.
- *Positive affirmations:* create positive, active, new statements about yourself as you would like to be: "I am relaxed. I am learning to express my feelings. I am expressing anger in a positive way. I am becoming more assertive. I am making realistic goals for myself. I am relaxing on my lunch break." Write out the statements and place them on your mirror, steering wheel, refrigerator, desk, or any place where they will catch your eye; repeat the statements to yourself several times daily. Be specific, positive, and brief.

4) **Learn Diaphragmatic breathing.** The diaphragm is the primary muscle involved in breathing. Most people waste effort by overusing muscles in the shoulders and chest to breathe. To practice diaphragmatic breathing, sit or recline in a comfortable position with legs uncrossed; place one hand on the chest and the other hand on the diaphragm, approximately two inches below the bottom center of the breastbone. Now practice breathing so that when you inhale the diaphragm expands; the hand covering the diaphragm moves out while the other hand remains almost still. As you exhale, the diaphragm relaxes and the hand covering it moves inward. Focus on *allowing* diaphragmatic breathing to occur rather than *trying*.

5) **Concentrate on allowing yourself (vs. trying) to cope with stress** and to relax; *trying* causes tension and can be avoided by an attitude of *letting* yourself relax, *allowing* yourself to be aware of your needs and wants, and by giving tender loving care to yourself.

6) **Seek work or tasks that you enjoy,** are capable of doing or learning, and which other people appreciate.

7) **Balance work and recreation**; learn to take relaxation breaks.
8) **Share feelings and concerns** with trusted friends, family members, or a counselor; let yourself become more aware of your feelings and express them to others in a positive way.
9) **Be a creative problem solver**; see NCPG #5:47, "Problem Solving."
10) **Avoid self-medication**. The ability to cope with stress comes from within you, not from the outside.
11) **Be aware of own energy and nutrition requirements.** Plan food intake to achieve and maintain ideal body weight with a well-balanced diet; see NCPG #5:41,"Diet: Weight Control."
12) **Learn to listen to your body** for messages of distress. Respond to early warning signals of tension or distress, using relaxation and creative problem solving.
13) **Set priorities;** take one thing at a time. Set limits in an assertive way; learn to say "no."

Teaching Objectives/Outcomes
1) Patient can identify own stress, stressors, and signs of distress.
2) Can describe stress syndrome and the relationship between chronic stress and chronic disease.
3) Can describe a plan to cope with stress in an adaptive way, including plan for exercise, relaxation, nutrition, problem solving, sharing feelings and concerns with trusted friend, family member, or counselor, and giving self tender loving care.

Recommended References
"A Code for Coping with Stress," by Hans Selye. *AORN Journal,* January 1977:35-42.
"Coping with Stress in Nursing," by M. Reres. *The American Nurse,* September 1977:4.
"Diet: Weight Control." *NCP Guide #5:41,* Nurseco, 1981.
Feeling Great: Images to Health and Well Being, by J. Segal. Santa Cruz: Unity Press, 1981.
Healing from Within, by Dennis Jaffee. New York: Alfred A. Knopf, 1980.
Mind as Healer, Mind as Slayer, by K. Pelletier. New York: Dell Publications, 1977.
"Problem Solving." *NCP Guide #5:47,* Nurseco, 1981.
The Relaxation Response, by H. Benson et al. New York: Wm. C. Morrow, 1975.
"Running for Life, Health and Pleasure," by B. Friedman and K. Knight. *The American Journal of Nursing,* April 1978:602-607.
"Stress and Coping: A Case for Intervention," by J. Scott. *The Journal of Psychiatric Nursing,* February 1977:14-17.
"Stress in Critically Ill Patients," by Carol A. Stephenson. *The American Journal of Nursing,* November 1977:1806-1808.
The Stress of Life, (Revised Ed.) by Hans Selye. New York: McGraw-Hill Book Co., 1976.
"Stress in the Surgical Patient," by M. Marcinek. *The American Journal of Nursing,* November 1977:1809-1811.
"Stressful Life Events and Coping Methods in Mental Illness and Wellness Behaviors," by J. Bell. *Nursing Research,* March 1977:136-141.

Tube Feedings: General Principles

GOAL: The patient maintains adequate nutrition via nasogastric or gastrostomy tube with safety and reasonable comfort.

General Considerations:
— **Purpose and Indications:** Enteral therapy via feeding tubes (nasogastric or gastrostomy) provides medication and liquid nutrition to meet the basic daily metabolic requirements for those patients who are unwilling or unable to swallow: patients who are in a debilitated, moribund, semi-comatose or comatose condition; or those with neurological impairment, disease, trauma or surgery of head, neck, oral structures or esophagus.
— **Types of Equipment and Supplies:** Formerly, large feeding tubes, size 14-18, were used to provide nutritional support. These were found to be associated with esophageal irritation, peptic esophagitis, upper gastrointestinal bleeding, and pressure necrosis. Now, smaller, size 6-8, softer, and more pliable feeding tubes are employed. Sometimes a stainless steel spring guide is inserted inside the small tube to facilitate passage. After the small tube is secured, the wire is slowly eased out of the feeding tube. See NCPG #5:46, "Nasogastric Intubation: General Principles."

  Commercial enteral therapy administration sets and gavage bags are available, but cheaper improvisations are still common: adapted enema bags, sterile plastic irrigation containers or resterilized IV bottles with IV administration sets. Electric volumetric or peristaltic pumps are sometimes needed to pressurize formula infusion through the smallest feeding tubes. For gastrostomy feedings, fifty milliliter piston syringes with Toomey adaptors or unbreakable ear syringes may be used to administer intermittent formula feeding.

  A wide variety of commercially prepared nutritional mixes are currently available, although blenderized food mixtures are still used at home and in many nursing homes. The needs of the patient for lactose-free, high-protein, low-residue, low-sodium or other type feedings are evaluted to prescribe the most appropriate liquid mixture.
— **Recommended methods and nursing responsibilities:** Initially, formulas are given half-strength and slowly (50 ml./hr.) to observe patient response. To be reported are nausea, vomiting, diarrhea, abdominal distention, cramping, allergic reactions, glucosuria, polyuria, or signs of fluid and electrolyte imbalance. After tolerance is assured, formula infusions are gradually increased to full strength at the desired rate and amount.

  Continuous drip infusions over 24-hour periods are sometimes advisable rather than intermittent feedings. Only a 4-8 hour formula supply should be hung at a time, and the container should be "time-taped" to help nurses keep feeding rate on schedule. Feedings should be stopped for at least thirty minutes before and after treatments such as physical therapy, pulmonary therapy, x-ray therapy or transfusions.

The gastric residual should be aspirated, measured and recorded before each intermittent feeding, whenever the patient complains of nausea, cramping or abdominal distention, and at least every two to four hours during continuous infusions. Report to the doctor delayed emptying of amounts greater than 150 ml. Reinstill up to 150 ml. of aspirated contents, then slow the formula infusion rate until further instructed. Getting the patient up in a chair or ambulating may help digestion.

Check infusion rate hourly and keep to appropriate rate. Do not attempt to "catch up" without specific orders to do so. Simply make a new "time-tape" for infusion container. Extracellular dehydration and osmolar overload can occur with patients who receive too much highly concentrated formula in too short a period of time. Observe for dry mouth, inelastic skin turgor or dryness of membranes, edema, fever, diminished responsiveness. Be aware of increased insensible fluid loss associated with high environmental heat and humidity. Note and report signs of thirst, polyuria, lethargy, copious respiratory secretions, and restlessness or pain.

Accurately record vital signs and blood pressure every eight hours, intake and output daily, and weight every other day. Check urine for sugar at least four times daily. Blood sugars are ordered for patients with glucosuria. In addition, periodic lab studies are needed to determine renal, hepatic, and hematologic function.

Good mouth care is essential. Have patient brush teeth and massage gums. Sucking on hard candy or gum chewing is sometimes permitted in alert patients to prevent dry mouth and parotitis. Gargles and mouth washes with warm saline should be done twice daily. Antiseptic or anesthetic sprays or lozenges may be prescribed for sore throat. Cream or ointment is applied to lips and nose to soothe dryness and irritation.

Provide explanations and support to patient, family, and friends as needed. Involve them in the feedings and care whenever appropriate. Listen to their questions and concerns.

Nursing Actions and General Principles of Tube Feedings:

1) Provide sufficient light, working space, and privacy so that nurse and patient can work together comfortably. Socialize with the patient and family as if this were a regular meal time. Joking about flavors, foods, and past dining experiences helps patient to cope with this adaptation of normal feeding pattern.

2) Arrange all necessary equipment and supplies in a readily accessible place to save time and energy. Keep them clean and covered between uses. Suggested items include:

- gavage administration set or substitute (asepto syringe, 50 ml. piston syringe with Toomey adaptor, or funnel),
- pitcher of water (room temperature) and an empty pitcher (for gastric residual),
- formula or liquid medication, (room temperature),
- tissues, towel or bed pad, and wet cloth for wiping up spills or leakage.

3) Elevate head of bed 30° and assist patient to a semi-Fowler's position.

4) Drape bed and patient near tube opening and feeding area.

5) Unclamp tube, attach barrel of syringe and aspirate gastric residual.

6) Measure gastric residual and re-administer if less than 150 ml. If amount is over 150 ml., re-administer only 150 ml., notify doctor and postpone tube feeding until further instructed.

7) Administer 30 ml. of water to clear tube, pinching off tube before it is empty. Add formula feeding gradually, raising or lowering tube as necessary to control flow rate so that infusion takes at least twenty minutes. Avoid instillation of air. Do not use force.

8) When prescribed amount is given, follow formula with 30-60 ml. water (20-25 ml. for a child). Clamp tube before entrance of tube empties of water. Rinse and insert catheter/tube plug into opening.

9) Leave head of bed elevated for at least an hour, but patient can be turned on right side and made comfortable or allowed to ambulate.

10) For gastrostomy tube feedings, cleanse skin area around tube opening. Apply protective skin ointment and fresh, dry sterile dressing. Secure tube.

11) Record patient response, time, amount of gastric residual, and amount of formula infusion.

Recommended References

"Effects of Diet Temperature on Tolerance of Enteral Feedings," by Karen S. Kagawa-Busby et al. *Nursing Research,* September/October 1980:276-280.

"Feeding Tube Introduction — An Easier Way," by E. Roblnson, Jr. and Paul Cox. *Critical Care Medicine,* August 1979:349.

"Fluid and Electrolyte Problems of Tube-Fed Patients," by Winifred Kubo et al. *The American Journal of Nursing,* June 1976:912-915.

"Giving Medications Through a Nasogastric Tube." *Nursing 80,* May 1980:71-73.

"Nasogastric Intubation: General Principles." *NCP Guide #5:46,* Nurseco, 1981.

"Update — Nasogastric Tube Feeding," by Barbara Griggs and Mary Hoppe. *The American Journal of Nursing,* March 1979:481-483.